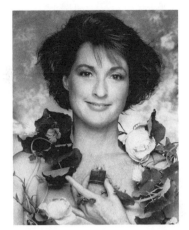

ABOUT THE AUTHOR

Alexandra Avery is a licensed Esthetician who has been researching and practicing natural approaches to skin care over the last twenty years. Alexandra believes that treating the skin with plant oils is a form of communion with Nature. She employs the healing and rejuvenating properties of plant essences to nourish, scent and preserve her formulas.

Alexandra developed a completely natural system of skin care products based on the purifying and nourishing essential oils used in ancient Egyptian cosmetics and mummification processes. Her family organic farm provides the herbal and floral base for her products.

At her Hawaiian health retreat, Alexandra personalizes skin care and body treatments for each guest. Alexandra Avery Purely Natural Body Care has received national awards for product purity and integrity. The line has consistently received top ratings in Shopping For A Better Planet, a consumers guide to conscious shopping. Alexandra especially enjoys speaking and writing on the benefits of Aromatherapy and natural skin care practices.

For more information on Alexandra Avery Purely Natural products or about her Hawaiian health retreat, please contact her through the Source Directory, page 116.

"The foundations of a civilization rest not in the mind but in the senses, and unless we can use the senses, we shall never have the biological conditions for human survival, let alone human progress."
Herbert Read

AUTHOR'S NOTE

As a child growing up on the shores of Hawaii, I spent many delighted hours hosting flower feasts with my friends, real and imaginary. Our home was flanked by Sea Heliotrope trees that lent themselves as spatial palaces, linked by intertwining branches and a few boards my father had put up. Beyond the tree forts, a bed of wild Woodrose vines stretched to the sandy beach and turquoise sea.

The preparations for these feasts were adventures that took me down the beach and into jungles of overgrowth. I collected the flowers that dreams are made of: Honeysuckle with its sweet stamens were my favorite treat. Red Hibiscus flowers became petal salad, with plump purple Sea Grapes served on the round flat leaves of the Sea Grape tree. The creamy whites of Jasmine, Gardenias, Wax flowers, Plumerias and Stephanotis (the traditional wedding flower) festooned the leafy roof. Our tea, oftentimes Kool-aid , was sipped from giant Cup of Golds, a plant with narcotic properties which probably added to our reverie.

There are a few memories of flower play that are not as pleasant, such as learning about the poisonous milk of the Plumeria tree. Although it was a lesson on flower power well learned, it was not a fun trip to the Doctors' office with threats of having my stomach pumped.

That experience pales however, next to the faux pas executed while learning about the plants in Minnesota. A crunch on a young Jack in the Pulpit bulb released a mouthful of oxalic acid which felt like hundreds of miniature pins in my tongue for hours afterward.

Such memories, both fond and otherwise, draw a history of my involvement with the plant kingdom, one which has led me along a beguilingly scented path. I have learned that there are many levels on which the flower essences work. It is my wish that flowers and their essences continue to help people discover their own unique rhythm with Nature, and through that relationship, to act with compassion and appreciation for all of life.

A Word About the Power of Essential Oils

Essential oils, like the plants they come from, may be dangerous if taken internally for too long a time. Therefore, although internal use of essential oils is a very effective means of treatment, it is recommended that you follow the applications as described in this book rather than adapt them for internal application.

I have made every effort to exclude any essential oils that are potentially toxic if taken internally or worn on the skin. It is your responsibility to treat and use the plants and their essences with respect for their value and potency. One way to determine the safety of an oil or formula on sensitive skin is to test patch an area of skin before using the formula on the overall body.

Be sure to keep all essential oils and dried plants in tightly closed bottles. All plant materials store best in cool, dark, dry areas. Essential oils will last years if kept under these optimum conditions.

Aromatherapy nourishes our bodies, minds and spirits in a vital, restorative way. Its benefits inspire celebration of our own essence and its' unique rhythm with nature. You can live as the flowers do, in a most creative expression of beauty!

Table of Contents

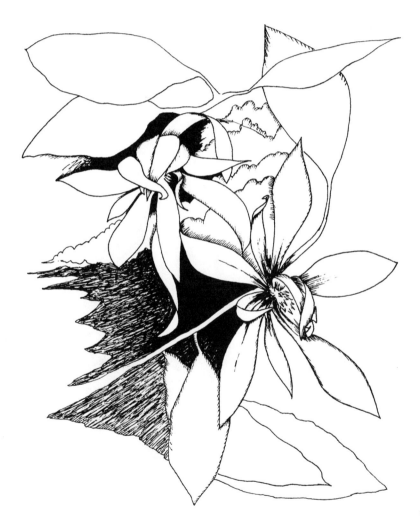

Ylang Ylang

PART 1

AROMATHERAPY

A RESPONSIBLE APPROACH TO NATURAL SKIN CARE

"The olfactory sense is an intricate part of everyday life. The moods you express are directly related to the fragrances surrounding you."

John E. Porter

AROMATHERAPY THEN AND NOW

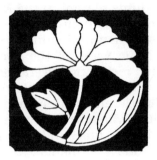

The art of Aromatherapy is not new to the world. The use of plants and their oils has been used to heal and beautify the body for over a hundred thousand years. Whether ingested, absorbed through the skin, or simply inhaled, plant aromas are known to have an effect on the body, mind, and emotions. Today, the study of aromas has been elevated to a science which employs the balancing and beautifying properties of pure herbal and floral essences to enhance the condition of the skin, body, hair, mind, and indeed, the environment.

Treatments with essential oils take many different forms. For centuries, Aromatherapy has been a part of Ayurvedic medicine. This is an Indian system which focuses on restoring the balance within the body, thereby promoting a healthful state of being. Since its first recorded use some 5,000 years ago, Ayurvedic medicine has been incorporating the healing powers of essential oils in candles, incense, massage oils. The Hindu doctors made extensive use of vaporizing various oils to soothe the skin and mind as well as to balance glandular functions.

In Egypt, oils were mixed with charcoal and ground herbs and pressed into small cone shapes which were worn inside men and women's hairpieces to scent the hair and relax the mind. It was the Egyptian priestesses and priests who extended the medicinal use of oils to the cosmetic use, creating a synthesis of inner and outer health and beauty. One of the most valuable contributions to future cultures

5

was their use of essential oils in embalming the dead, the very same oils that were used to rejuvenate and soften the skin! Many beautifying treatments were practiced by the Egyptian people, and their association of medicine and cosmetics remained popular well into the Middle Ages.

The art of perfumery was pioneered by an Arabian Doctor named Avicenna. His discovery of oil distillation led to the opening of the perfume market in the Middle East. At the same time, the Chinese were practicing with many aromatics, combining Aromatherapy treatments with Acupuncture.

During the plague years of the Middle Ages, lockets containing aromatic restoratives were worn by women and men. It was during this time that western medical practitioners began to realize the antiseptic potency of many essential oils. Many Herbalists who relied on these essential oils were able to keep their health intact and were later burned at the stake for sharing this information. Oils were infused in vinegars and drunk, as they still are today, to maintain and improve health.

Many Roman and French leaders left legends of voracious use of aromatics, both for healing and pleasurable purposes. In ancient Rome streets were lined with rose petals to celebrate the arrival of certain leaders.

In France, Louis XIV became known as the "sweetest smelling monarch" and would have the water in the Versailles fountains replaced with perfume for special occasions. His successor, Louis XV had a different scent designated for each day of the year and the cost of scents used by his mistress, Madame de Pompadour, constituted the largest household expense. Napoleon was a lover of Spanish Jasmine, splashing himself with over 60 flasks a month. He is known to have emptied entire bottles over his head to revitalize himself on the battlefield!

The person who coined the term Aromatherapy was the French chemist Rene Maurice Gattefosse who experimented intensely with flower essences and their medicinal uses. He was particularly instrumental in the development of our understanding of the antiseptic uses of oils. It was Gattefosse who discovered the healing effects of Lavender on burns. When working in his laboratory one day he severely burned his hand. A vat of Lavender oil was near and he plunged his hand into it. The healing was remarkably quick and led him to working more extensively with the Lavender herb.

Aromatherapists, people employing the healing and beautifying properties of aromas, have use of over 400 essential oils in their treatments. These oils may be extracted from the roots, leaves, resins, bark, flowers, seeds, or the rinds of fruits. An important part of Aromatherapy is that many essential oils enhance relaxation so that one is able to concentrate in a more perceptive and positive mode.

Different persons may react differently to different aromas, especially in dealing with conditions of the mind. Robert B. Tisserand, author of The Art of Aromatherapy, explains: "Each essence has its own personality, its own set of attributes, and this can be used to bring out certain qualities in us; helping us to see ourselves more clearly, to understand our faults, and to let the beauty and joy of our souls breathe a fresh, summery fragrance through our minds."

Cosmetic Aromatherapy deals with the face and body in particular, and the mind and emotions as secondary, though no less important effects. The molecular composition of the essences allow them to easily penetrate the skin, helping to stimulate circulation, lymph flow, and the detoxification and revitalization of the cells.

The heating and cooling powers of essential oils assist in regulating the proper circulation to and from cell tissues. First, cells receive a good supply of oxygen and nutrition essential to cell function. Secondly, the return circulation is improved, cleansing the cell of the wastes created during cell metabolism. This oxygenating and detoxifying power of essential oils aids in hydrating the tissues and maintaining optimal capillary action and vitality to the tissue.

The molecules of essential oils are small enough to penetrate the skin's outer layers. This allows for rapid penetration into the skin, and makes essential oils efficient carriers for other ingredients in natural cosmetics. How deep into the lower layers they go is the subject of current research.

Research is proving that the natural preservation properties of essential oils have a life extension effect on skin cells. Most essential oils have strong bactericidal and fungicidal properties, without the weakening and depleting side effects of synthetic antibiotics. It has been demonstrated over the years that essential oils are effective against almost all pathogenic bacteria occurring in infectious diseases. Rather than weakening the immune system as do many conventional drugs, Aromatherapy has the ability to stimulate and strengthen the immune system.

7

It is hard to keep up with advances in the field of skin care because what is promised tomorrow is quickly becoming today's beauty regimen. Science has shown us that skin is more renewable, penetrable, and resilient than previously thought. In addition to confirming our faith in the many beauty benefits that Nature provides, we are also seeing an explosion of high-tech products on the cosmetic counters across the country.

Researchers in Denmark have reportedly found a protein that rejuvenates human skin in cell cultures. This protein supposedly reverses the aging of the skin cell. When skin cells are young they have a small distinct nucleus and are bound together by smooth strands of protein. As cells age they lose their smoothness and elasticity, becoming flaccid, with a large, fuzzy nucleus. The proteins that bind the cells to one another break down, causing room for wrinkles to form. This protein miracle is called Factor X, and the exact origin and nature remains a secret until approved and patented. Clinical trials of Factor X in skin creams are under way in Europe, and if all goes well, the mysterious Factor X will be available on the market in a few years.

Many botanical or plant extracts that have been popular over the last decade are now receiving attention from the skin care researchers. Studies are isolating the elements and compounds of many herbs (some single extracts can have as many as 50-100 elements, each with a different activity) and for the first time, scientifically measuring the benefits that have been known to practitioners for literally thousands of years.

Some of the most noted herbs being studied are the anti-inflammatory and anti-irritants such as Chamomile, Horse Chestnut, St. John's Wort, and Aloe Vera. Arnica, a potent little white flower, is being studied for its skin firming ability.

For years the beauty industry has been making all sorts of claims about products, many of which have not been scientifically established. The gap between product advertising and actual skin enhancement is beginning to close. There is even talk among manufacturers to regulate these claims, since no two companies perform tests in exactly the same way. We will be seeing standards for how product tests are to be conducted.

Skin care developments and medical science will be more closely aligned in the 90's. The big cosmetic firms are turning to larger and better research departments in an effort to bridge the gap between the FDA Drug Act and the Cosmetic

Act. We can look forward to more accurate lists of ingredients on labels though the understanding of the increasingly complex designer chemicals will still rest on the consumer.

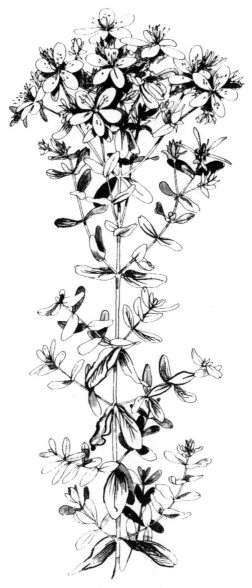

St. John'sWort

DEVELOPING THE SCIENCE OF FLOWERS

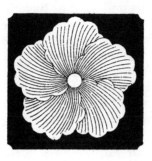

Most people are surprised to learn that our sense of smell is 10,000 times more sensitive than our sense of taste. Our olfactory system may even contain more receptor cells than the eyes. The sense of smell has the most direct and expedient connection to the brain of all the five senses.

When inhaling a flower or an essential oil, scent molecules are received immediately within the brain via the smell receptors or olfactory nerves at the back of the nasal cavity. The scent is then registered within the limbic system, the most primitive part of the brain. Here lies the seat of our emotions, our memory, the base of our learning ability, and the regulator of sensory motor activities. Research has shown that we can have a physiological response to odor.

Olfactory science, the study of smell, is a rising star in the field of human research. There are an estimated 500,000 scents to distinguish on our planet, each described mainly through associations with something else. There is a very limited vocabulary when it comes to describing odors in a basic sense. Unlike sight and sound, it is difficult to measure smell. In vision one can refer to a rainbow of color; in sound, one relates to sound frequencies. The sense of smell has no spectrum to which one can refer.

The study of smells is of great benefit to science today. Many scientific centers have conducted tests to show that certain odors produce mood changes, a belief that has been held by Aromatherapy practitioners for centuries. In such past studies, brain-wave machines were connected to people, measuring the effects of a variety of odors, and examining a specific type of brain-wave activity that is very sensitive to changes in mood. These objective measurements were studied along with psychological mood-mapping techniques which rely on the person's subjective evaluation of scents.

Psycho-Aromatherapy is opening up new measures for the human mind. Related studies have worked with cancer patients, using positively associated smells, to counteract negative associations with chemotherapy treatments. A Duke University Medical School experiment has determined that the sense of smell is responsible for triggering the rise of a natural biochemical called histamine when a person smells a food to which she/he has a known allergy.

Research is showing that women have a greater proclivity toward scent identification and association than do men. Tests have shown that, although the scent-color association appears to be a learned response, women have an easier time drawing connections between scent and color (i.e.: the smell of Lemon to yellow).

It is now known that some diseases such as Alzheimer's cause smelling deficiencies, and diabetes causes body odors. In this time of immune deficiency disorders, doctors and researchers are aligning the sense of smell with the immune system. "There is some belief that the sense of smell is the external version of the immune system, that by smelling certain things, there's actually a connection to the immune system that produces the necessary reaction antibodies to counter it." (Dr. Tom Orofino, William H, Wheeler Center for Odor Research, Chattanooga, TN.)

Research companies are jumping on the bandwagon to cut and protect their piece of the fragrant pie. After a study found that muscle tension and blood pressure were lowered after inhaling an apple spice blend containing Nutmeg oil, IFF sought and received a patent on the use of Nutmeg as a stress reducing odorant. Could that have been the secret in mom's good old fashioned apple pie?

By the end of this decade, the psychological effects of smells will be setting the mood in many unexpected places. Imagine an environmental system diffusing relaxing aromas in city subways, mind alerting aromas in truckers' cabs. These research efforts are being applied in state and private ventures around the world: a calming cedar smell effuses through a large public rest stop on a Japanese highway and this same system is now operating in some U.S. hotels.

Calming fragrances are also being used in many work places with beneficial results. In a Japanese study, a soothing lemon fragrance was wafted throughout a factory of video terminal operators for one month, and the worker's error rate dropped in half. Researchers theorized that the calming scent helped to diffuse a high-tension environment.

Will mood altering scents become the Muzak of the 90's, improving lives by enhancing alertness, productivity, relaxation, and more? In an era where perfume and fragrances have been sold for personal aesthetics alone, we are now discovering a new and even more valuable aspect of fragrance, its' functional and therapeutic benefits. This is not entirely surprising to those who remember the days of smelling salts (the ammonia compound stimulates the terminal nerve, relieving a fainting victim).

Environment plays an important ally (and sometimes adversary) to our sense of smell. Almost all of the products we use in the bathroom, kitchen, office and household in general are perfumed. There are many odors that can be perceived even when diluted billions and trillions of times. Our olfactory sense is almost continually barraged with a myriad of scents, and desensitization of the sense of smell can occur with over- stimulation of scents.

There are few who have not experienced the onslaught of an over scented environment. Most cosmetics have fragrances that consist of 50 to 150 chemicals. The average person uses about 12 different cosmetic products daily. That amounts to a large arsenal of chemicals barraging the skin and senses on a daily basis.

Many essences in cosmetic formulations are derived from natural sources but are broken down and processed to such an extent that they end up with few or no signs of the important original properties. One of the most important distinctions in Aromatherapy is that the essences used must be of natural origin to be of complete benefit to the body and mind. That is, the essences must be from plants rather than synthetically reproduced from plant origin.

It is easier for the body to absorb and utilize aromas when they are pure, natural substances inhaled, worn, or ingested. I have found the effects of the active plant ingredients to be a gentle and powerful opening to a greater awareness of my own physical, mental and emotional capabilities.

THE POLITICS OF BEAUTY

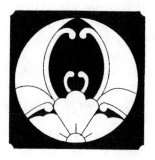

Cosmetics have come a long way from the days in which they were first created, when the Egyptians blended healing unguents and potions from the finest herbs and oils. Today, Americans spend close to $3 billion annually on cosmetics for the face and body. There is an astonishingly slick industry of advertising behind todays' cosmetic manufacturers, bent more toward 'sales at whatever cost' rather than education of the consumer.

The packaging and advertising do more in determining the cost of the product than do the ingredients. Have you noticed how most mass marketed cosmetics advertise their products behind a veil of mystery, sensual secrecy, and little if no ingredient listings?

A favorite tactic of cosmetic advertisers is to lend a buzz word such as collagen, protein, anti-aging, or natural to the ad, when the product in mention has very little to do with the words advertisers know will grab attention. It is left up to the consumer to differentiate between ingredient listings and to determine the short and long term effects of such cosmetics.

We have been manipulated into thinking that higher priced mass marketed cosmetics contain the better ingredients. The truth is that the cost is set by the marketing departments, not by the cost of ingredients. Particularly with perfumes, the price is often 20 times the cost of the product. Of course the advertising and packaging help to sell cosmetics: we know that a purchase is decided upon within a few seconds of viewing the product by most consumers. But do we want to pay more for the evocative advertising and sumptuous packaging than we do for the product itself? To this issue the American consumer is beginning to "just say NO!"

The natural cosmetics industry has gained a great deal of ground in the last decade, as people look toward a more safe, gentle, and ecological approach to skin and body care. Most natural cosmetic companies spend advertising dollars on educating the consumer rather than promoting an image, because they believe the consumer wants to take more responsibility for her/his personal welfare.

The trend of modern beauty is now encompassing the whole person, rather than simply 'looking good'. The natural cosmetic industry has helped to balance this concept of beauty, bringing inner health and beauty to the surface. In a sense, we are renewing the ancient Egyptian approach to cosmetics, both a healing and beautifying treatment. The Egyptian embalmers brought to light some of the best ingredients for healing, soothing and rejuvenating the skin: resins and oils that are used in some of the best natural cosmetics available today.

BEAUTY
WITHOUT THE BEAST

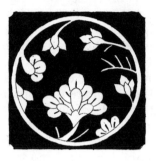

All of the chemicals that could possibly be used in manufacturing body care products have already been tested, so why do companies continually retest? Many do so as a matter or course, testing and retesting every batch of cream even though there are no variations whatsoever in the formula. It is distressing to think that these companies continue to test on animals in order to satisfy insurance requirements for company protection.

Of the eight standard whole animal toxicity tests, there are three main tests given to animals in cosmetic Labs. They are the Draize Skin Irritant Test, the Draize Eye Irritant Test, and the LD 50 test. The Draize Skin-Irritant Test is performed on rabbits. This experiment determines the amount of irritation caused by a particular substance when applied directly to the rabbits skin. Preparations for the test include shaving and abrading the skin. Concentrated doses of product chemicals are necessary, and the amount of tissue damage over a given period of time determines the efficacy of the product for human use. The rabbits experience anything from mild redness and swelling to death.

Another standard procedure is the LD 50 ("lethal dose 50%") test. This measures the amount of a specific substance required to kill half a group of animals, hence LD 50. Although scientists agree that this procedure provides little useful information about potential health risks to humans, it continues to be a common practice in many cosmetic companies. Even though many industry scientists have publicly stated that it is difficult, if not impossible, to use animal data to determine the effects on humans, millions of animals continue to suffer under the guise of product safety.

Many years of hard campaigning on the behalf of animals rights have brought some positive changes in the cosmetic industry. The new wave of cruelty free shoppers is making an impact on the big business of cosmetics. More and more shoppers are making a conscientious effort to buy cosmetics and household products that contain environmentally sound ingredients, that are not tested on animals, and that contain no animal by-products. We the consumers can enhance the ethical integrity of the skin care industry and help create a more compassionate quality of life.

Several major cosmetic companies have ended years of animal testing and many others are considering alternatives to animal testing. Many have enacted temporary moratoriums on animal testing but continue to buy raw ingredients from manufacturers who may do live animal testing. Proposals to limit or ban animal tests are being introduced on both federal and state levels as Humane Cosmetics move into the mainstream market.

The Cosmetic, Toiletry and Fragrance Association, the industry's chief trade organization, has contributed funds toward research on more humane testing procedures. Research into alternatives to the LD 50 test has come up with several more humane procedures. Modified LD 50s, using fewer animals, could reduce animal deaths by 90%. There is at present no other officially accepted replacement to the Draize Eye-Irritancy Test. Alternative methods involving chicken egg membranes, cell cultures, and invertebrates have potential to replace living mammals in product safety tests. Computer models and in vitro tissue cultures may eventually replace animals altogether.

Animal Rights Actions You Can Take

1. Refuse to purchase products that have been manufactured and marketed by subjecting animals to toxicity tests.

2. Help educate others about unnecessary product safety tests for cosmetics. The Humane Society of the U.S. sells bumper stickers saying, "Do Something Beautiful-Buy Cruelty-Free Cosmetics" for $.50. See address below.

3. Send your contribution to the Humane Society of the US (HSUS) to continue their efforts to eliminate unnecessary animal testing. Now that they have prompted cosmetic companies to develop alternatives, we must all work toward convincing them to implement these non-animal tests! Write to: HSUS 2100 L STREET NW, Washington DC 20037. (202) 452-1100.

4. Write to the Cosmetic, Toiletry and Fragrance Association (CTFA) urging it to increase financial support for the development and implementation of non-animal testing methods. Write to: CTFA 1110 VERMONT AVE., NW, SUITE 800, WASHINGTON DC 20005.

5. Write to the FDA, the regulatory agency which does NOT require animal tests to determine product safety of cosmetics. Urge the FDA not to accept data from the Classical LD 50 test. This would result in the industry's adopting alternative testing methods. Write to: Food and Drug Administration, Cosmetics Division, 200 C Street SW, Washington DC 20024.

6. Send donations to the American fund for Alternatives to Animal Research, 175 W. 12th St. #16, New York, NY 10011-8275. This group of researchers and educators has contributed greatly to the Animal Rights movement.

7. The MOVEMENT ACTION PLAN is a valuable tool providing activists with a practical, how-to-do-it tool for organizing and instigating social movements. Send $2.00 for information to Social Movement Empowerment Project, 721 Shrader St., San Francisco, CA 94117. (415) 387-3361.

8. People for The Ethical Treatment of Animals (PETA) has a catalog of cruelty free products for personal, home and office use. It lists companies that do animal testing so that you can make wiser consumer choices. P.O. Box 42516, Washington DC 20015. (301)770 PETA.

BEAUTY AND THE ENVIRONMENT

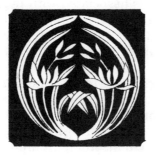

One can hardly make a commitment to a cruelty free personal care regime without also considering our environmental responsibilities. As planetary citizens we have the honor and responsibility to care for the planet in every little way we are capable. It is empowering to include the welfare of the environment in every day considerations!

There is a wealth of information already available on recycling. Find out your towns' recycling network and practice a conservation of consumption. Commit yourself to recycle and re-use as much a possible. Choose products packaged in recyclable material. Avoid buying over-packaged products.

Be aware of products and ingredients that are harmful to the environment and exclude them from your shopping. This is a big responsibility because it requires investigation, alertness and a truly compassionate heart. Learn ways in which you and your shopping dollars can help protect our environment.

There are hundreds of cosmetic grade chemicals that cause damage to our bodies and the environment. Among them are a large number of ingredients that are banned in other countries but allowed in American cosmetics. Of 2,750 cosmetic ingredients reviewed by the U.S. General Accounting Office, 600 were found toxic, including 125 known carcinogens, 26 causing birth defects, and 20 causing nervous system disorders. The same report stated that "manu-

21

facturers do not have to determine the safety for their products before selling them . . . as a result, hazardous cosmetics can be marketed until the FDA obtains information to prove the product may be injurious to users."

Did you know that the snow white facial tissues, toilet paper and cotton balls used in your daily personal care regime may be a threat to your health? We've all grown up thinking that white is associated with hygiene. These pure white products pose a threat not only to our health but to our environment as well! The chlorination process in paper mills produces Dioxin, one of the most lethal of man made chemicals.

Dioxin is the term used to describe a group of 75 similar compounds, all highly toxic. The most deadly in the group is compared to plutonium. Minute quantities cause health effects such as strong headaches, insomnia, hair loss, aching joints, immune system disorders, reproductive failure, and birth defects. Dioxin is highly bioaccumulative. It is stored in the fat cells and is found in the milk of North American mothers.

Since the North American pulp and paper industry has not been pressured by the EPA to revise its noxious processing, it is up to the consumer to change the demand for bleached paper products. Your responsibility can then become to shop for recycled, chlorine-free and/or unbleached paper products.

What about the safety of the products applied with your pure or not-so-pure white tissues? Of the 4,000 ingredients that go into cosmetic formulations, you can bet there are some that are hazardous! There are safe alternatives to every toxic ingredient and they are expertly lined out in the Medical Self-Care Book of Women's Health by Bobbie Hasselbring. Many toxic cosmetic ingredients and common irritants have been identified, "blue dye #1, P-hydroxyanisole, triethanolamine (TEA), diethanolamine (DEA), iron oxides, EDTA, BHT, PVP, lead acetate, toluene, phenol, and sodium saccharin."

It is of vital importance to read labels and make responsible decisions concerning ingredient listings on cosmetic containers. We are no longer in an age where we have the luxury of saving just our own skins; we now must turn our attention to the environment with the same zeal that the fitness craze turned toward our bodies.

Requesting businesses to use recycled products will encourage manufacturers to improve their methods. Every ton of recycled paper saves about seventeen trees, eliminates 70 per cent of air pollutants, 50 per cent of water pollutants and more than three cubic yards of landfill space.

This is the decade of planetary responsibility. How can you contribute toward a more humane and ecologically balanced planet? Your stand will make a difference. Start in your own home and with your friends. Contact community and national environmental interest groups to find out how to become more involved. See the recommended reading section.

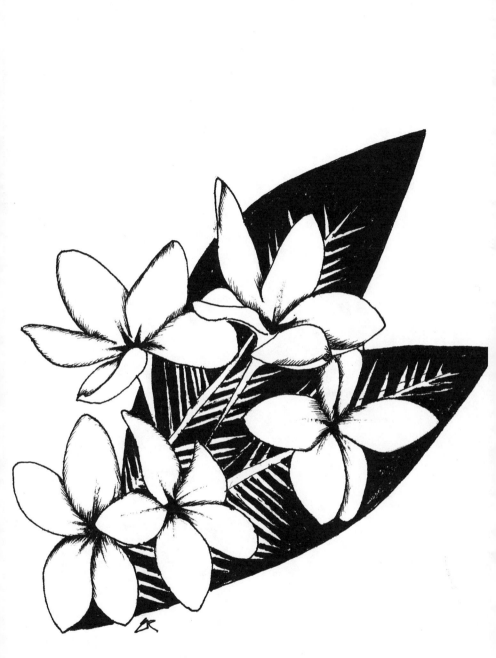

Plumeria

PART II

THE AESTHETIC VIEW

"The sense of smell is the most cerebral of our senses. Lost memory can be immediately reclaimed through the recognitive powers of smell. The sense of smell is discreet, setting a mood quietly and unobtrusively. The sense of smell is therapeutic, becoming increasingly important to the maintenance of our physical and mental well being"

Laura Bellows

YOUR SKIN
A CLOSE UP LOOK

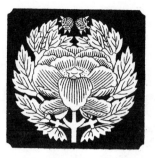

The skin is the body's largest organ, and next to the brain, the most important. It measures approximately 20 square feet and weighs between 7 and 9 pounds, twice as much as the brain. It requires one third of the body's circulatory blood for healthy functioning.

The skin is often referred to as the third kidney because of its eliminative role. Skin excretes up to two pounds of waste daily, moving more toxins than all the eliminative organs combined.

The skin's main release of toxins is through perspiration. This function assists in regulating body temperature and PH balance. It also is a way to burn a few calories, approximately 500 per day. When perspiration is inhibited, the kidneys pick up the responsibility for eliminating the waste, and the body risks being subjected to a toxic state. The skin most often ends up with the telltale sign (blemishes result as the skin attempts to eliminate the toxic accumulations in the blood.

In addition to its most important eliminative function, the skin performs six other basic functions.

1. It is a protective barrier from heat, cold, bacteria and other environmental stresses.

2. It regulates the body temperature, maintaining its inside temperature despite wide variations on the outside of the skin.

3. It breathes to a small extent, exhaling carbon dioxide and eliminating unwanted gases.

4. It absorbs substances, passing them through the tissues.

5. It has its own hydration system which keeps it soft and supple, and lubricates itself by discharging the sebaceous fluids through perspiration.

6. It contains a complex networking of nerve endings that allow us sensation and enable us to react to heat, cold, pain and pleasure.

Most people begin to pay more attention to their skin when the effects of aging are first noticed, generally between the ages of twenty and thirty. By the beginning of the next century there will be approximately 32 million Americans over the age of 65. With increasing life spans, there is a natural increase in skin care and a healthy life-style. This chapter will give you facts about what the skin is and what happens to it as we age.

The skin is made up of three main layers: epidermis, dermis, and subcutis. Each of these layers support the other and has its own particular function. All of these layers are made up of cells in varying degrees of life potency. Of the some hundred trillion cells in the body, we shed up to five billion a day! Without being too technical, following is a concise explanation of how these layers function and interact in normal, healthy skin.

EPIDERMIS LAYER

The epidermis is the uppermost layer of skin, composing of fifteen to twenty overlapping layers. This part of the skin contains no blood vessels, but has many small nerve endings. The Stratum Corneum, also called the Horny layer, is the outermost layer. Its cells are tightly compacted, tough, and scaly like the horn of an animal. Keratin, which forms our horny layer is the same protein material that forms horns in mammals. These cells remain on the surface for about two weeks and are shed as new cells from underneath come to the surface. When these cells do not slough off normally , a dull, flaky complexion results. The Horny layer serves a most important function. Being the main physical barrier to the environment, it shields against environmental sub-stances, including some of the sun's harmful ultraviolet rays.

These overlapping cells are covered by a thin layer of oil called the Acid Mantle which helps the outer layer to retain moisture. The acid mantle of the skin is a natural acidic covering over the top layer, protecting us against bacterial build-up. It is made up primarily of lactic acid and sodium salt mixed with the oil gland secretions, called sebaceous fluids. For most individuals under normal conditions, the acid mantle will range between 4.5 and 5.5.

In addition to the acid mantle, the outer layer contains natural chemicals that also aid in maintaining the moisture balance of the skin. These constituents are commonly referred to as the Natural Moisturizing Factor (NMF) which contains amino acids, minerals, salts, and urea (a cellular waste product) as the main ingredients.

When we maintain the NMF and the acid mantle, our skin retains a soft, moist and supple appearance. Many factors contribute to the demise of this balance, among them sun damage, an unhealthy diet, and incorrect cleansing regimes, such as regular use of soap which destroys the acid mantle.

The middle and thickest layer of the epidermis is called the Stratum Spinosum. It is made up of irregularly shaped cells This is where cell division occurs, the new cells being constantly pushed upwards toward the skin surface. As these cells progress toward the outer layer, they flatten out, lose their water content and begin to die. This process takes from 15 to 25 days depending on the age and health of the person.

When one looks at the skin anthropomorphically, this outer layer of skin corresponds to the outer layer or skin of plants. The most widely used of these in skin care are the oils of the skin or rind of citrus, specifically Orange and Lemon. These oils are used topically to strengthen the outer layer of skin, strengthen the skin flora and the acid mantle, strengthen hair and nails, increase tissue regeneration, as well as soften the skin.

DERMIS LAYER

The dermis is where the major effects of the aging process take place. It is made up of fibrous connective tissues. The tissues contain collagen protein and elastin fibers which support the epidermis and give the skin its elastic quality.

The Dermis also houses minute sensory nerve endings to alert the mind to temperature changes, pressure, pleasure and pain. There are numerous capillaries, veins and arteries which branch from larger vessels within the body. In fact, every square inch of Dermis contains up to fifteen feet of these tiny blood vessels. These vessels carry nutrients and provide oxygenation as well as remove metabolic waste materials. There is also a supply of the melanin skin pigment in this layer.

Underneath these tissues is the deepest layer of dermis, the reticular layer, home of numerous blood vessels, sweat glands, oil glands, nerves, lymph vessels, hair follicles and the arrector pili muscles which are minute involuntary muscle fibers inserted into the bases of the hair follicles.

This middle section of the skin is best complemented with leaf oils. Pine, Peppermint, Rosemary, Lavender, Thyme, Sage all assist the functions of the dermis layer. These essential oils stimulate blood and lymph circulation, detoxify skin tissues, promote healthy secretion of the tissues, tightens fibers of the connective tissues and increases the skin metabolism.

SUBCUTANEOUS LAYER

Below the Dermis is the fatty Subcutaneous layer of tissue. This is the cushion for the skin, giving smoothness and contour to the body. Its cushioning value varies according to the age, sex (women start with more) and general health of each person. This fatty layer also stores reserve energy for the body.

This layer is responsible for the deposit of fat molecules, promoting circulation, energy and heat discharge, and to some degree, tightening of the connective tissue. The essential oils most beneficial to this layer are the root oils of the plant. This is the layer of skin where regeneration first takes place. The oils related to the regeneration organs of the body are Sandalwood with its androgen stimulators, Terragon and Vetiver with their estrogen stimulators.

SKIN STRUCTURE

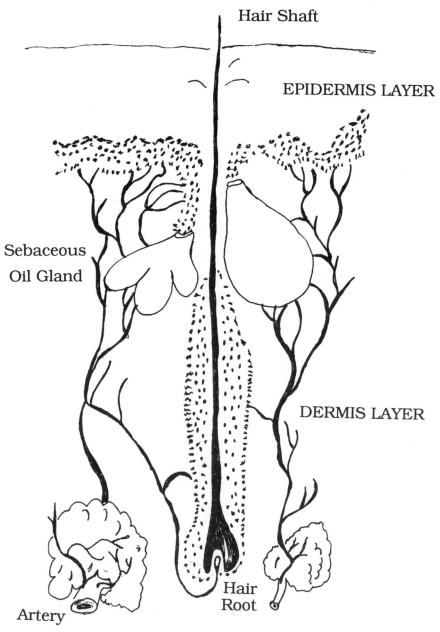

Hair Shaft

EPIDERMIS LAYER

Sebaceous
Oil Gland

DERMIS LAYER

Hair
Root

Artery

SUBCUTANEOUS LAYER

SKIN TYPES AND THEIR AROMATHERAPY VALUES

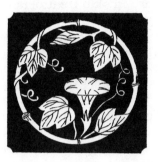

As a skin care researcher and Esthetician, I have seen a wide variety of skin conditions and types. The structure of each person's skin is basically the same though its function varies depending on one's health and environment. For instance, in my Hawaii practice, I see a majority of dry, dehydrated faces. In Oregon (the rain state) I work with more supple-skinned faces because of the greater moisture (and less sun) factor.

Not only does the environment play a major role in optimum skin integrity, but the functions of the various systems involved also plays a key role in skin health. Both the blood and lymph systems must be taken into account as well, for a healthy skin is a well nourished skin, and the nourishment essentially comes from these two systems.

Biological programming, our heredity, is probably the most influential factor in determining our skin type. It has been medically demonstrated that the balance of male and female hormones affects the production of the sebaceous glands. More sebum is stimulated by male hormones, meaning, according to medical research, that men have a greater tendency toward oily skin. Skin on the scalp, face, back and chest contains more oil glands than skin on the arms and legs.

The activity of the sebaceous glands does decrease as we age, gradually changing an oily complexion to a drier skin. This process is speeded up by medical complications, some medications, or certain skin treatments. A woman who has recently had a hysterectomy, a menopausal woman, or a person undergoing chemotherapy will most often experience a change in skin type.

It is probable that a person will experience many skin conditions in a lifetime, since the skin is a constant reflection of our age and inner well-being. One's skin condition varies on a daily basis depending on temperature, humidity, travel factors (airplane air is drying to the skin, different water sources interact differently with the skin), exercise, and outdoor exposure.

A description of each type and the Aromatherapy applications for each type are meant to provide you with a basic outline. It is important to correctly evaluate your skin type so that your treatment of it will appropriately correspond.

The skin surface can be divided into four basic groups:

SENSITIVE

UNDERACTIVE

ACTIVE

OVERACTIVE

SENSITIVE

Sensitive skin is delicate, generally light in color and tone, and when treated correctly, reflects a porcelain glow and fineness. It is almost always dry skin. It is easily irritated and should be treated with very mild, non detergent products. Both fragrances and preservatives can cause reactions and such products should first be patch tested on a less sensitive part of the body.

Sensitive skin is generally a thin textured skin, making capillaries, or blood vessels more visible. Because the blood supply is generally closer to the surface of the skin, it is more prone to irritations or allergies. In some cases, the tiny blood vessels, being so close to the surface, are damaged by environmental stresses. They rupture, creating a condition called cuperose, which most often occurs over the cheeks and across the nose. Alcohol consumption, spicy foods, and increased blood flow through exercise and even blushing, can contribute to cuperose problems.

This skin type can react unfavorably to many synthetic chemicals in skin care products. In addition, environmental stresses such as excessive heat and cold, wind, and exposure to ultraviolet light increase the aging process by damaging delicate tissues.

Aromatherapy Choices for Sensitive skin

It is best to avoid using strong soaps, alcohols, and synthetic colorings, fragrances or preservatives on the skin.

1. Jasmine - Soothing, emollient, skin softening.

2. Neroli - Reduces inflammation, regenerates skin cells.

3. Chamomile - Reduces inflammation, calms the skin.

4. Rose - Hydrating, emollient, calming, can help diminish enlarged capillaries.

5. Frankincense - Anti-inflammatory, prevents wrinkling.

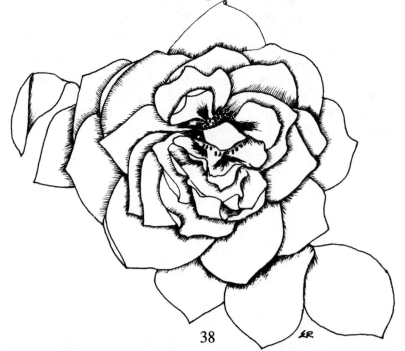

UNDERACTIVE

Underactive skin is found most commonly on a fair skin that easily burns in the sun. It is often sensitive with a somewhat delicate texture, poor elasticity, and generally lacks tone and suppleness. It does not commonly break out in blemishes or acne, but has an all over taut feeling, sometimes showing signs of flaking or peeling. Flakiness is a sign of dehydration. Sebum production is somewhat sparse or impaired, resulting in moisture loss which increases the tendency toward wrinkling and fine lines, particularly around the mouth and eyes.

I like to refer to dry or underactive skin as a need for stimulation of the various layers. The treatment of dry skin necessitates increasing the blood circulation which is a primary factor in plumping and regenerating skin tissue. The easiest way to accomplish this yourself, without electronic equipment, is through massage.

Since water comprises about 70% of the constituents of the skin, it is understandable that the skin serves as a sort of reservoir for the rest of the body. It is widely confirmed that a relative humidity of 60-65% helps to maintain the skins natural moisture content. A lower relative humidity draws moisture from the skin into the environment, and a higher relative humidity forces moisture into the skin. Hydrate the skin with a rich moisturizer both morning and night, using a moisture replenishing toner spray between times.

Aromatherapy choices for Underactive skin

Calendula oil is added to the base oils. It helps the formation of new skin tissue, and has a mildly stimulating effect on underlying blood flow, helping to speed waste removal in tissues and provides essential nutrients to tissues.

1. Orange Blossom - Balances dry skin, increases cell regeneration.

2. Italian Jasmine - Skin softening and moisture replenishing.

3. Rosemary - Stimulating, rejuvenating, tonic.

4. Myrrh - Stimulant, helps skin exfoliation, antiseptic.

5. Sandalwood - Antiseptic, hydrates and softens skin.

Rosemary

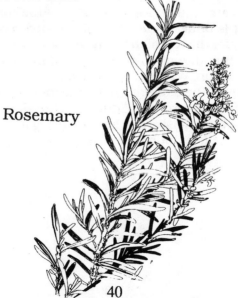

ACTIVE SKIN

Active skin is most often seen in glamor magazines models who are pre-adolescent. Truly, it is not the most common skin type, and is found mainly in young and/or health oriented individuals. Active skin shows a normal function of the body's organs and systems, a good balance of oil and moisture, a general sign of good health, physically, mentally, and emotionally. It most often has a firm, supple and smooth appearance.

Most people have a combination skin type, recognized by an oilier T zone (forehead, nose and chin) with a drier look around the cheek, jaw and hairline. It is really two different types of skin, and should be treated accordingly. The aim is to moisturize the dry areas and stabilize the more oily areas.

This skin type is also classified as Active/Underactive skin. Use a combination of the Active skin treatment on the oilier areas and the Underactive treatment on the drier areas.

Aromatherapy choices for Active skin

1. Lavender - Soothes skin, balances sebaceous glands, stimulates cell regeneration.

2. Rose Geranium - Astringent, cleansing,
   humectant, rejuvenates.

3. Neroli - Antiseptic, reduces inflammation, skin cell rejuvenate.

4. Clary Sage - Stimulates cellular regeneration, hydrating.

5. Patchouli - Mild bactericide, mild skin
   tonic, cleansing.

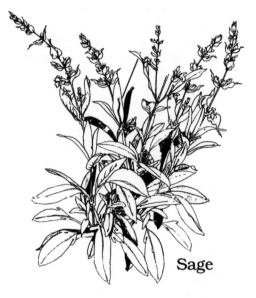

Sage

OVERACTIVE SKIN

Overactive skin is often a strong hereditary trait. The most commonly identifiable characteristic is an all over shiny look from the oil secretions which are heaviest in the T zone. A thick skin texture with large pores, particularly around the nose area, are signs of overactive skin. Because of the pronounced sebaceous activity, this skin type will appear smoother and more plump than Underactive skin. This excessive oil production will keep a face looking more youthful much longer than a dry skin type.

Bacteria from one's fingertips and the environment at large tend to breed in the oily film which contains toxic wastes from the body. Although oily skin is prone to developing acne in younger persons, other factors beside oily skin are also responsible. Stress, improper cleansing, poor diet, hormonal imbalance, heredity and nervous habits contribute to skin eruptions.

Acne is a chronic inflammation of the sebaceous gland and hair follicle, and most types can be treated with proper home care. Bacteria within the hair follicle multiply approximately every half hour, and when the follicle becomes blocked, acne or pus formation rapidly develops. In severe conditions such as acne cysts, it is advisable to have the skin examined by a dermatologist before embarking on your own treatment program. Most cases of skin eruptions and acne involve a disturbed PH balance in the skin. In this case the skin is over acetic, with a higher PH than normal. Because acne is a disease of the skin tissue it is very important to treat it appropriately. I recommend that the Aromatherapeutic treatment be a step toward treating this disease but not the only approach. It is extremely important to follow the strictest hygiene practices.

Aromatherapy choices for Overactive Skin

1. Rose Geranium - Highly antiseptic, used for many skin diseases.

2. Ylang Ylang - Soothing to oily skin.

3. Niaouli - Strong antiseptic, helps heal skin eruptions.

4. Lemon - Controls sebaceous activity, cleansing, tightens open pores, anti-wrinkle properties.

5. Lavender - Controls bacteria, oily skin, acne, eczema.

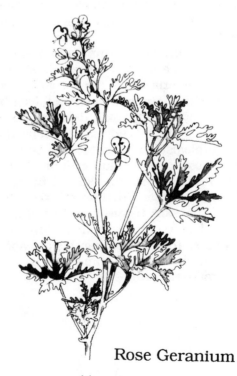

Rose Geranium

THE AROMATIC FACIAL

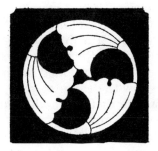

One of the great pleasures of an Aromatherapy facial is, of course, the scents. One drop is enough to evoke a fragrant journey as far as your imagination can travel. Scent triggers the memory, so your journeys may take you to past events that had been otherwise unnoticed in the memory bank.

During one of my Aromatherapy facials I was reminded of an experience that I had forgotten. It was the Pine scent that carried me back to the Oahu north shore forests where, as a Brownie scout, I had gone on a hiking adventure with my troop. Pine forests are not a significant part of the Hawaiian terrain, but there were a few Pine and Eucalyptus trees along our path. I believe it was the first time I had smelled the pungent Pine and Eucalyptus scent in nature. What came back to me was that the hike turned into a quest for the Pupukea Man, the island's equivalent of Big Foot. All of a sudden I could recall the sheer excitement we felt in our search for clues, a sighting, and the shared thoughts of befriending this mythical beast. The recalled feeling of sacred adventure, the thrill of possibly bringing fantasy face to face with reality flooded the moment with a sense of magic.

When working with essential oils, it is imperative to use an eyedropper because no personal formula will contain more that 10 drops of oil. It is equally important to keep oils stored in small bottles. Any air space, even in a small amber bottle, is an invitation for oil oxidation, which will shorten the life span of your oil. If you are storing them in eyedropper bottles, be sure that your bottle remains upright. Most essential oils react with rubber, eventually breaking down the rubber and creating a mess, not to mention changing the quality of your oil.

For convenience, I made a fabric pouch with little pockets to store my aromas. It is easy to carry around, keeps the tiny oil bottles separated and safe from breakage, and allows no light to reach the bottles. I keep a couple of eyedroppers in the pouch with a 1 ounce bottle of my favorite oil blend which I refill as necessary. Such a precious bag deserves to go everywhere: simply inhale the scents from the bottles or use them in any of the ways mentioned in The Aromatic Body.

Before you begin with designing your own facial system, take a good look at your diet to see what adjustments may be necessary to provide your body with the best nutrition possible. Consider ways in which you can approach stress reduction. Take stock of the products you currently use on your skin. Is there a more humane and environmentally responsible approach you can take? Are the ingredients in your products nutritional, or is the ingredient list merely an economic consideration for the manufacturer; a list of inexpensive fillers and extenders equivalent to a refined food such as fluffy white bread?

Since your pores are absorbing what you put on your skin, thus entering the tissues and to some extent, the blood, doesn't it make sense that you would want to use the same quality on your body as you ingest in your body? Why make your body work extra to try to rid itself of non-assimilable ingredients that will otherwise hang out in the body as debris and potential toxins.

You will want to create an ambiance of relaxation while giving yourself or your friend a facial. All of the mood enhancers play well with Aromatherapy: Scented candles can be made by lightly rubbing them with a few drops of essential oil. Pleasurable music enhances auditory relaxation. My favorite facials are given to the natural sounds of the ocean waves and the cooing of doves in the softly blowing palm trees.

Soft, clean washcloths and face towel and a comfortable massage table or bed to rest on offer a luxurious pampering. About an hour of time will be sufficient to complete your aromatic facial.

The six simple steps to your home facial

For each of these steps you can create your own personalized Aromatherapy approach.

Cleanse

Exfoliate

Steam and pore cleansing

Massage

Mask

Moisturize

STEP 1: CLEANSE

Whether you use a cleansing cream, cleansing milk, or a mild soap cleanser, your procedure will be the same. You can add 4 drops of your scent blend to every 2 ounces of any product on hand, unless it is already an Aromatherapy product.

Moisten hands, spread about a teaspoon of product over fingertips, and apply to face and neck. Start at the chin, sweep outward to the end of the jaw. With a continual stroke, draw the fingers in to the base of the nose, up to the temple, down along the side of the nose, up over the bridge of the nose, between the brows, and across the forehead to the temples. Work in under the eyes toward the bridge of the nose, and out across the eyelids. with a little more product, make upward strokes on the neck and throat area.

The small, upward, circular movements of the fingertips will gently stimulate the skin and help to emulsify any surface debris.

Remove product with a warm, damp wash cloth or face towel. Start at the neck and work upwards. If you are also removing eye makeup, you may want to wipe it off first with a damp cotton pad. (It is best to avoid paper tissue since the wood fibers may cause minute scratches on the skin surface, inviting places for bacteria to breed.) Continue the cleansing with a tone dampened cotton pad. You can save money on cotton pads by separating a pad into two once it is wetted with the toner.

STEP 2: EXFOLIATE

This step includes removing dead skin cells that the cleansing has softened and loosened. It refines the texture of the skin, leaving it with a smoother and fresher look. Our bodies daily shed billions of cells, and when encouraging this process, the skin retains a more healthful glow.

Select which essential oils you want to use according to your skin type. Add three to five drops of your blend to one of the exfoliant formulas in Recipes For Rejuvenation. You may want to add the drops to a product you have found really works for you. The drier or more sensitive skin types will require the most delicate treatment in exfoliating dead skin.

Mix the oils with the exfoliant just before applying to face and neck. Most exfoliating products are applied to the skin, massaged in, and rinsed off. Some are left on for five to ten minutes. For those types of exfoliants, I prefer to brush it on with a flat watercolor brush, though fingers or a thin facial sponge work.

To remove exfoliant, use a gentle brushing with a soft complexion brush, facial sponge, or soft cotton wash cloth. An oily, thicker skin type will respond to a more vigorous brushing of the skin. The motion is the same for all skin types, small circular motions, concentrating around the nose and where clogged pores are present.

It is best to avoid using products with ground shells in them unless they are very finely ground. The coarse edges of the nut shell pieces can cut the skin, leaving it looking red (sometimes mistaken for a healthy glow) and feeling tender or warm.

STEP 3 : STEAM

If you are using the easy pot method, heat 1 quart of water to boiling. Add 4-6 drops of your chosen essential oil. Wrap your hair in a towel if you want it to stay dry and out of the way. When the water begins to boil, remove pot from stove. Sit comfortably over the pot and make a tent over your head and pot with a towel. Take long, deep, slow breaths. Your exhalations will stir the steam, creating little blasts of warmth. For a cleansing and relaxing treatment, 3-5 minutes is sufficient, though 5 minutes affords a deeper cleansing.

Another quick and easy way to steam the face is to wrap the face in warm, moist hand towels. Fill the basin or a large bowl with very warm water, Add 3 drops of Ylang Ylang oil for a wonderfully relaxing effect. Fold the hand towel in half, lengthwise, and dip it into the basin of water. Wring out the towel and fold it around the face, leaving a hole over the mouth and the nostrils. You may want to repeat this once or twice in order to adequately steam the face. the towels cool off rather quickly.

An Epi-sauna or facial steaming device is a wonderful and fairly inexpensive appliance to have on hand. Fill the receptacle with water and herbal material plus 5 drops of essential oil. Set the steamer up so that you can sit comfortably during your steaming.

My preferred method of steaming is with a hand held Lucas steamer. This is a most thorough method because the steam is pressurized and gently penetrates the pores, affording a deep cleansing. The gentle pressure of the steam helps added essential oils to be absorbed at the deepest level of skin tissue possible. It is especially good for dry, sensitive and mature skin types because the steam is not hot. I have used this little French machine (it is somewhat reminiscent of an espresso machine) for 15 years. I have taken mine with me to deserts where it becomes my portable rainforest. Fill the receptacle 1/4 full of distilled water, 3/4 full of toner, and add 5 drops of desired essential oils. Spray the face and neck, using light sweeping movements to aid in penetration.

PORE CLEANSING

Before doing any kind of extraction, dab the area with some toner or a disencrustant solution. A disencrustant softens the debris in the pores, making their extraction easier.

It is very important to observe the most sterile conditions possible when removing debris or hardened oils from the pores. Wrap each index finger in a thin layer of astringent soaked cotton or gauze. Make sure you have a well lit area around your mirror. What you want to do is to keep one finger still, and with the pad of the other finger, use a gentle milking action to press the debris from the pore. Dab the area with an astringent containing an antiseptic oil such as Cedar or Sandalwood.

It is important to stress that there are some skin eruptions only a qualified esthetician or dermatologist should tend to. If you have frequent eruptions, and you have corrected your diet and stress patterns, it is my recommendation that you consult a professional .

STEP 4: MASSAGE

The facial massage comprises about 1/4 of your facial time, and is definitely the most relaxing 10 to 15 minutes of your facial. A facial massage can be done daily or several times a week as a skin toning and strengthening practice.

There are a lot of tiny lymph vessels in the face and neck. Proper massage technique helps to drain the excess lymph and remove internal debris and toxins from the head.

Manual stimulation of the facial muscles tones and rejuvenates the skin tissues, bringing increased circulation and nerve supply to the face. Relaxation and decreased stress are other rewards of massage.

Refer to the Facial Massage Techniques and chart for an understanding on how to massage the face. Even a shortened version, when applying your night moisturizer, is beneficial to the skin.

STEP 5: MASK

There are many benefits of a facial mask. It increases blood circulation in the areas covered, absorbs and removes excess surface oil, removes surface dirt and skin debris and softens and smooths the skin. Masks are refreshing, relaxing and they firm the skin, improving the skin tone.

One fun thing about masks is that there are so many different kinds to make. I have given you formulas for my favorites and hope they will interest you in experimenting with your own concoctions.

There are two basic groups that masks fall into, the drawing masks and the treatment masks. Drawing masks are made from clay or mud, and have definite drawing ability. Treatment masks and moisture packs help to seal in moisture, holding it in the top layer of the skin. The skin plumps with the extra moisture and conditioning ingredients, thinning out the lines for a short period of time.

Since a clay based mask completes the deep cleansing by absorbing and drawing residual wastes and bacteria from the pores, it is good to include some clay in most masks. A clay based mask can be used regularly on normal to oily skin types. Because a clay mask also draws some excess oil from the skin, it is best to alternate it with a moisture pack when giving facials to dry or sensitive skin types.

This is the part of the facial when Aromatherapy has the most time to work on the skin. The aromas I have listed aid in skin cell regeneration by stimulating the circulation and providing emollients to deeply moisturize.

Sensitive skin can be tricky to work with at this step. If you have sensitive skin, it is best to experiment with the essential oils, one at a time, so that you know how each oil feels on your skin before you make an aromatherapeutic combination. If you experience any kind of itching or burning, you may have used too many drops of essential oil, or you may be reacting to the oil or some other ingredient in the mask. Remove the mask, splash cool water on the face, and wait ten minutes before applying any moisturizer. This will give your skin time to re-balance itself.

When applying the mask, stand over a basin so that if it drips you will not have to worry about clean up. Start with the neck and brush (you may also use you fingers but the brush will apply it more evenly) upward, covering all areas except the lips and around the eyes. With any left over mask you can paint your upper chest area or refrigerate it in a tightly closed container. Most masks will last for up to one week.

Take a cotton pad with toner on it, divide the layers to make two pads, and place them over you eyes once you have found a resting spot. I love to briefly soak the pads in a few tablespoons of water with 3 drops of Chamomile Blue. Azulen, the blue coloration in Chamomile, is both softening and anti-inflammatory. You may want to apply some moisturizer under the eye area during this time. For the next 10-15 minutes, allow yourself the pleasure of deeply relaxing. This is a time to think of all your tensions being released, pulled out of the body just as the unwanted waste is being pulled from the pores.

To remove the mask, dip the face towel into the basin of scented water, and wrap the face again to re-moisten the mask. This will make it easier to remove. Using the face towel or your cosmetic sponges, gently dab your face with warm water until the mask is removed. Splash your face with cool water, mist liberally with toner, and let your face air dry. The skin will absorb this moisture and it will help to draw in the moisturizer.

STEP 6: MOISTURIZE

A good moisturizer provides nourishment and a protective shield over the top layer of skin. The massage action of applying the cream stimulates the blood supply which assists in skin tone improvement. Since the skin is nourished from the blood and lymphatic vessels, absorption of your moisturizer affects the cells locally, and through the blood and lymph systems, the whole metabolism of the body as well.

There are three types of moisturizers: an oil base for normal to dry types, a water based for oily and acne types and a gel based moisturizer. All oil and water based creams are emulsions, or blends of the two ingredients. Most water based creams are mainly just that, water. We know that water is a very good humectant, or moisture attracting agent, but why spend a lot of money on a product that is primarily water? Check your ingredient listing to see how much water you are buying. The ingredients are listed in the order of their quantity in the formula, most to least. Likewise, you should know what the ingredients themselves are. What you put on your face really ought to be of the same quality as what you put in your mouth, don't you think?

The moisturizing massage can be done in a very short time. Use even and light motions, and be careful not to drag the skin by pulling or stretching it. Begin by covering each fingertip with a small amount of cream.

-Using gentle upward strokes, smooth your fingertips up the neck toward the chin.

-Move from the center of the chin to the front of the ears, moving up the cheek in this manner.

-With the index fingers, start at the center of the lower lip, stroking around the mouth, up over the upper lip, and stop at the nose.

-Gently draw the index and middle fingers down the bridge of the nose and out across the cheekbone to the temple.

-With a little more cream on the fingertips, if necessary, begin circling the eyes from the temple toward the inside corner and out over the eyelids, using a light patting motion.

-Circle the eye, ending at the bridge of the nose this time, then smooth fingers straight up to the hairline, and out across the forehead. Repeat this motion while moving down the forehead.

YOUR PERSONALIZED FACIAL

Your personalized facial will be determined mainly by your current skin condition and type. In addition, you may create specific aromatherapy combinations to enhance or change your mental and emotional well being.

There are several ways in which essential oils may be incorporated into each phase of your daily skin care regime: cleansing, toning, and moisturizing. It is best to make up small batches of treatments until you decide on the best individual or combination for your own skin. You'll need a glass bottle with eyedropper lid to store the essential oil combination. Make sure, of course, that you are working with pure plant essences and not synthetic blends.

The most enjoyable facials I've ever had were at the beach in Hawaii, given in love and fun with my women friends. The Mermaid Mask has become a regular routine at the beach. I mix the powdered ingredients with sea water. When the mask has dried, I take a long swim while the mask dissolves back into the ocean.

Here are ways in which you can make your current skin care regime a most aromatic and healthful pleasure:

CLEANSING

If you use a cleansing milk, add 5 drops per 4 oz. bottle of cleanser. If you want to make one of our cleansers, follow the instructions as given and add your own Aromatherapy blend instead of any aromas listed in the formula. Use the same amount of your blend as suggested in the formula.

TONING

Even if you have oily or overactive skin, make sure your toner or astringent does not contain alcohol. Witch hazel is far superior to alcohol, which causes excessive drying to the tissues. To every 4 ounces of toner, add 5-8 drops of your oil combination. Make sure to vigorously shake the bottle before each use in order to completely distribute the oils throughout the toner. Use the toner on cotton or from an atomizer. I carry a spray bottle in my bag and another in my car so that I am never without a hydrating misting during the day.

MOISTURIZING

A very simple and most effective body moisturizer can easily be made and kept on hand for morning and evening moisture replenishing effective on all skin types. Combine equal amounts of Apricot Kernel, Sweet Almond and Wheat Germ oil. These vegetable oils are easily absorbed and are rich in Vitamins A, B, D, and E. To each ounce of this blend add 15 drops of your specific aromatherapeutic blend. This moisture rich blend can be used on the body as well as the face, remembering that a little goes a long way. It is best to apply the oil to the body when it is still slightly damp from the shower or bath. The water on the skin helps increase the absorption rate into the tissues.

Your Aromatherapy skin care regime will produce positive results with a minimum of effort and time. Your skin will not only look better, you will feel the effects of the aromatics through renewed energy, heightened libido, uplifted moods, and a sense of overall balance.

FACIAL MASSAGE TECHNIQUES

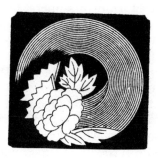

Massage dates back to the Greeks who used it as a cure for ailments. The term is derived from the Arabic word "massa" meaning "to touch" or "to stroke." There are many forms of massage today. The technique I have used over the last 15 years is a combination of basic massage strokes with a Chinese system of healing called Acupressure.

This is a very important part of the facial because the massage stimulates the blood circulation, relaxes tense muscles, strengthens weak muscle tissue, stimulates glandular activity and stimulates the nerves. The skin exhibits noticeable results from a massage. There is a fresh color to the face, a more vibrant and healthy glow. The muscles, as they relax, lend a softer look to the face.

The areas of massage are the forehead, cheeks, lips, eyes, and neck. The following page shows a diagram of the facial muscles. It is a good idea to become familiar with the main muscle groups, and where the muscles originate. The correct way to massage the muscles is toward their origin.

Acupressure, as with massage, encourages the body's own natural balance. Both support the underlying muscle tissue, and the increased circulation restores the skin tissues, bringing nutrients and vitality to plump the tissues. The acupressure points relate to various organs and areas of the body. It is the same system as acupuncture, only the tools are your fingertips rather than needles. The points are located by feeling for slight cup shaped depressions just under the skin surface. The pressure is gentle but steady, applied for one minute to each point.

Rather than cover the entire system of acupressure in detail, I will focus on the most important points relating to facial toning. For a more complete understanding of this ancient system of healing, I recommend the books by Irma Teegarten, a woman who has spent her life teaching this system. There are many schools of acupressure that base their programs on her teachings.

The massage is done just before the mask so you can take advantage of the increased circulation. The nutrients in the mask will be more easily absorbed and utilized. After your facial, it is ideal to allow your face to rest for a good hour before doing any heavy exercise, and if you wear make-up, before applying makeup. This gives the pores some time to finish closing. Some of the moisturizer will be exhaled by the pores during this time. Any makeup applied may have a shiny or slightly greasy appearance from the cream residue.

The massage may be done daily, in either its full form or a shortened version, as described in the moisturizing section. I prefer to take time at the end of the day to do my daily facial massage, sometimes when I get into bed before falling to sleep. This helps to relieve muscle strain or tension from the days activities, as well as to nourish the nerves and facial tissues. You may want to use the mirror until you are more familiar with what you are doing.

Start by putting half a teaspoon of your selected Aromatherapy facial oil into the palm of your hand. Briefly rub your hands together to warm the oil a little. Cover your face with the palms of your hands, eyes closed, and take a few deep breaths. Inhale and exhale slowly. The Aromatherapy treatment has begun. Your mind as well as your skin responds immediately.

FOREHEAD

Interlock the fingers of each hand over the middle of the forehead. Slide the fingers, with slight pressure, toward the temples. At the temples, rotate fingertips in an upward and outward motion. Repeat several times. Starting at the brow line, rotate fingers in the same way out to the hairline. Move up the forehead in rows of these rotating movements.

Two fingers width above the center of the eyebrows you'll feel an indented acupressure point. Make small inward circles on this point. This has an effect on headaches and insomnia. The last point is directly above the eyes, at the hairline. Make small inward circles using firm pressure.

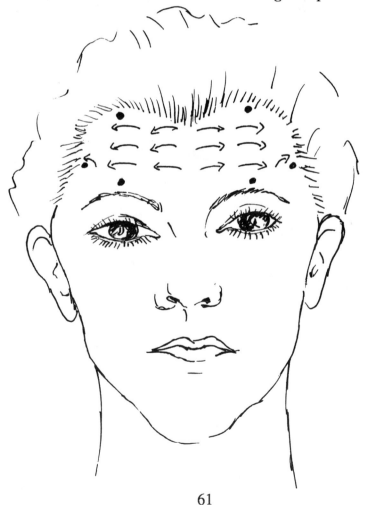

EYES

Circle the eyes, moving out over the brow and gently in toward the bridge of the nose. Repeat each stop three times. Stop at the outer end of the eyebrows, and press in small outward circles. Remember to feel for the slight indentation of the acupressure point. This point stimulates the muscles, helping to tone the tissue under which crow-feet wrinkles develop. Do the same at the outside corners of your eyes. You will be pressing on the socket bone ridge, not the eyeball itself.

Now take the eyebrows between the thumbs and index fingers, and pinch them together, moving along the length of the brow. Smooth the eye area with gentle strokes over the eyes to the temples. Rotate the fingers around the temples with moderate pressure.

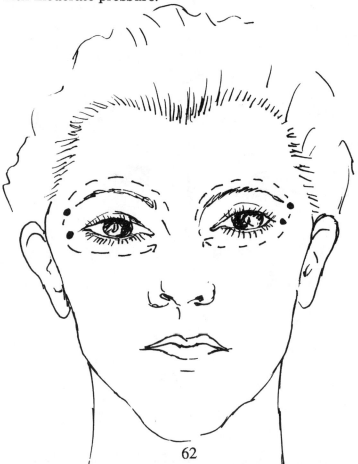

CHEEKS

Start with the third and fourth fingertips at the bridge of the nose. With fingertips spread slightly apart, slide across the cheeks to the hairline. Continue this motion 5 or 6 times. Stop at the junction where the jaw hinges together. Gently but firmly press in small outward circles. This is an important acupressure point, as it brings energy into the entire face. Repeat threee times.

Two finger widths away from the nostrils is another acupressure point. Press upward into the undersides of the cheekbone, making small outward circles. The increased circulation will bring a rosy glow to the cheeks. Repeat three times.

NOSE

Bring the middle finges up the sides of the nose to the top of the bridge. Press upward, making small inward circles on the bone. Traditionally, this point is pressed to relieve eyestrain, headache and sinus congestion.

Press the middle fingers down the sides of the nose making little outward circles. At the base of the nose, beside each nostril, press and hold for 10 seconds. This acupuncture point corresponds to the lungs. Take a few slow deep breaths through the nose, exhaling through the mouth. Shake your hands a bit, add a little more oil if necessary, and close your eyes. With eyes closed, look down and out toward the top of the cheekbones. This is very restful for the eyes. You will notice a sense of opening and relaxing in the middle of the face where so much tension gathers.

MOUTH AND JAW

Move from the mouth to the middle of the ears pressing with the fingertips. Repeat three times. Find the pressure point between the chin and the lower lip, about half an inch from the corners of your mouth. Press firmly in small outward circles. Next, take the lips between the thumbs and index fingers, and squeeze them together, holding for 30 seconds. Lightly tap around the mouth to stimulate the area. With small outward circles, press the acupressure points above your upper lip, about half an inch from the corners of the mouth.

Massage under the jaw line by gently lifting with the tips of the fingers and slide back toward the ears. Repeat several times. With the backs of the fingers, make little rhythmic slaps just below the chin. The stimulation of the slapping will help to firm this fleshy area.

Start tapping the face with the fingertips. This stimulating motion improves circulation, enhancing cell growth. Spend a little extra tapping time around the mouth and under the chin where skin generally needs the most toning. There are a lot of lymph nodes just under the chin. Massaging these with gentle circular motions will increase the lymph drainage from the area.

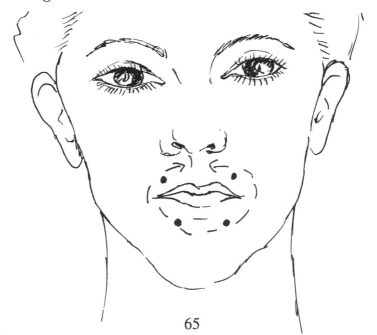

NECK

Draw the hands down to the base of the neck. Slowly slide the fingers, one after the other, up the neck to the chin line. Use slightly heavier pressure on the sides of the neck. You may notice some tenderness on the sides of the neck. The lymph glands, when congested, will be tender and sometimes feel swollen. Massage this area with moderate pressure to stimulate the lymph flow. With one index finger, press firmly on the groove of the bone at the base of your throat. The pressure should be downward, not inward.

FACIAL EXERCISES: A NONSURGICAL FACE LIFT

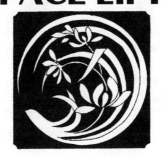

Tired of that "thinker's line" between your brows? Bothered by the drooping look at the corners of your mouth? These and other facial lines can be improved over time with correct exercising of the muscles beneath them. The muscles of the face, neck and head, when exercised in a controlled manner, will be richly nourished by the blood circulation, resulting in increased tone and contour of the skin. They can also be trained to control unwanted or unattractive facial expressions. Facial beauty is directly related to the level of tension in the head and neck muscles. Tension in these areas can restrict the blood circulation, increasing general stress throughout the body.

There are a number of different facial exercise systems to promote and maintain facial tone and contour. Below is an easy method of seven simple exercises, which when done daily for just a week, will open you to a new awareness of your facial structure. To train the muscles and to achieve control over your facial expressions, it will be necessary to regularly and correctly practice the exercises. It is best to do each exercise seven times, seven times a week for seven weeks. After that, taper off to three times a week to maintain control of the muscles involved.

An ideal time to practice the exercises is after you have moisturized your face each night. To begin, pull your hair away from your face. You want to be able to observe your entire face in a mirror. Apply a rich moisturizer over the face. Sit comfortably in front of a mirror. Begin the seven steps.

SEVEN STEP FACIAL EXERCISE

1. Relax the mouth and jaw, letting the jaw hang but keeping the mouth closed. Lips should be soft, not tensed. Moving only the corners of the mouth, slowly raise them toward the temples. Do not let forehead move even though it will want to. Very slowly, raise the corners as far as they will go, then, just as slowly release the muscles until the mouth returns to resting position. The object is deliberate, slow and controlled movements.

2. Open the mouth slightly, keeping the lips relaxed. Slowly pull up on the skin of the nose, as though wrinkling it. Hold it in that position while you repeat the first exercise. Slowly release nose and mouth together.

3. Let eyelids partially close, looking up and toward the middle of the forehead. Slowly raise the lower eyelid in and upward, until you feel a slight strain, then return to the beginning position.

4. You will be repeating the last exercise and adding some resistance to encourage the muscles to work more deeply. Relax and drop the jaw, opening the mouth to an oval shape. Press your index finger into the chin for some support.

5. This is difficult to get the hang of, but you will feel it from the chin down to the lower neck when done correctly. Push the jaw and lower teeth out and up over the upper teeth and lip. Without any movement in your lips, push the chin muscles up as high as you can. Your chin muscles are doing all the work. Your forehead, as before, remains still.

6. With thumbs facing outward, place your fists under the chin. Press up with your hands as you push down with your head. Hold for the count of three and repeat three times.

7. Now you get to move the forehead while keeping the rest of the face stationary. To prevent the eyebrows from lifting, firmly cover them with your index fingers. Lift the forehead muscles up and back. You are working beneath the skin surface really; the forehead skin should not crinkle. Relax forehead, and keeping fingers on brows, repeat the exercise.

ACUPUNCTURE FACIAL TONING

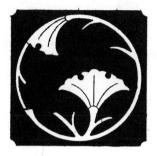

I have been a believer of acupuncture since the day I got over my fear of needles, the day of my first acupuncture treatment. I have experienced the toning and balancing effects of Chinese herbs and acupuncture and have seen many dramatic recoveries using this approach.

Acupuncture can be very effective in reducing lines and wrinkles in the face, chin and neck. It can tighten the skin around the eyes, mouth and other areas of the face. Acupuncture needles stimulate the 30 muscles under the facial skin, tightening them and minimizing the depth of facial lines. A balancing to the energy patterns flowing through the face and body leaves one feeling very refreshed and restored.

Optimum treatment sessions are twice weekly for approximately ten consecutive sessions. Depending on the acupuncturist, treatments usually cost between $35-$60. Follow up treatments may be recommended every six months.

When Dr. Karl Toubman told me about his work with acupuncture facial toning, I immediately signed myself and my husband up for a series of 10. My husband received treatments twice weekly and I received them weekly. Although he is 6 years older than I and makes his living outdoors under blistering skies, his results were more noticeable much more immediate than mine. His squint lines around his eyes were noticeably reduced after three sessions.

There was a firmer feeling of the skin, and a healthy glow noticeable after each treatment. I experienced the same positive effects even though it seemed to take longer for my skin to improve. I notice a more vibrant skin tone and a more even coloring. The lines on my forehead, around my mouth and eyes are definitely minimized. My conclusion after the ten sessions is that I would rather use this approach for a year or two than to facial surgery in order to minimize wrinkles and increase the youthful appearance of my skin.

For more information about facial toning with acupuncture, contact a certified Acupuncturist in your town or write to Dr. Karl Toubman at P.O. Box 2744 Kamuela, Hawaii 96743.

SUPPLEMENTING SKIN VITALITY

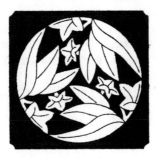

There are easy ways to keep the skin in a glowing healthy state. Drink a half-gallon of water a day. Eat a balanced diet with lots of vegetables, whole grains and fresh fruits. Steam or sauna your skin on a regular basis. Exercise moderately. Quit or reduce smoking, caffeine and alcohol consumption. Keep a positive attitude and live a fulfilling life-style. In addition, herbal and vitamin supplements may be helpful. Following is a brief description of the vitamins most beneficial to the skin.

VITAMIN E

Remember slathering vitamin E all over your face, despite claims from the medical establishment that it not only fails as a rejuvenate for the skin but that it does nothing for the sex-drive either? Since its discovery in the 1920's, vitamin E has been subjected to a great deal of controversial research. Now, scientists are preparing to show how vitamin E, the great anti-oxidant, has an anti-wrinkling effect when applied topically.

"The presence of adequate vitamin E is necessary for the efficient use of oxygen in the tissues," cites J.G. Hellstrom in his report of vitamin E and its role in healing wounds. Vitamin E fights free radicals, the wild molecules that the skin creates in fighting pollution and ultraviolet light. Be-

71

cause of its known penetration value, vitamin E moisturizes the skin assisting in the maintenance of connective tissue.

Vitamin E has been shown to strengthen antibody formation, and its effect on reducing the incidences of cancer is under current investigation. There have been extensive studies of topically applied vitamin E over the years. In addition to skin moisturization, it has shown to significantly aid in the treatment of chronic skin diseases, wound healing, scar reduction and acts as an anti-inflammatory.

Foods rich in vitamin E are Wheat germ, Sesame seeds, Sunflower seeds, and all natural grain cereals.

VITAMIN C

Vitamin C is finally getting its due attention and claim. Linus Pauling put up with the taunts of the medical establishment for his research on vitamin C for over 30 years. Now, in addition to the general acceptance of vitamin C as a cold fighter, we know that it also increases collagen production. Because vitamin C is water soluble, it is not easily absorbed into the skin. Methods of topical absorption are under study, and we can look forward to another natural remedy for lines and wrinkles in the near future. This will be especially beneficial to people with thin skin, because it will mean eventual thicker skin.

A deficiency of vitamin C in the body will contribute to cellular breakdown, and over a period of years, will speed up the aging process. Smokers deplete their body of up to 150 mg. of C with each cigarette inhaled.

Foods rich in vitamin C are Apples, Bananas, Beets, Cabbage, Grapefruit, raw green vegetables, Kale, Lemons, Oranges, Peaches, Pineapples, Parsley, Papayas, Sprouts, Raspberries, Strawberries, Tomatoes, Watercress.

VITAMIN A

Perhaps the greatest vitamin discovery in skin care is that of vitamin A. Topical benefits of this skin vitamin include improved water barrier properties of the skin, speeded wound healing, improved cell development, and anti-keratinizing (protecting the skin from the formation of crusty patches of skin cells.) It also helps the skin and mucus membranes resist infection.

Vitamin A betacarotene is the pigment giving many foods an orange-yellow color: Cantaloupe, Carrots, Sweet potatoes, Squashes. Chemical derivatives of vitamin A, retinoids, have been compounded into a variety of products to treat everything from acne to psoriasis. Retinoids became a household word with the discovery that Retin-A banishes wrinkles as well as acne. Retinoid therapy and related drugs are a popular mainstream method of treatment for acne, uneven skin tone due to pregnancy or sun-exposure, and even hair loss. See next chapter on Skin, Stress, and Sun.

Foods high in vitamin A are Apricots, Carrots, hot red peppers, Kale, Sweet potatoes, Spinach, Turnips, Beet greens, Squash, Cantaloupe, Broccoli, dried Prunes, and Lettuce.

VITAMIN B

The B vitamin family is an important group for skin care. Most notably is B 2 or riboflavin, which helps keep the skin clear and smooth. **Sources are Milk, Cheese, Fish, Egg yolk, Bran, Molasses, Wheat germ, Liver, and lean meats.** Niacin contributes to healthy skin, assisting the body in using oxygen to make energy from the food ingested. **Sources of niacin include whole grains, dried Beans, Peas, Peanuts, and lean meats.**

VITAMIN D

It is hard to talk about the skin and omit the importance of vitamin D, the sun vitamin. Then again, it is hard for me to talk about the sun and its effects on the skin because, having grown up in the tropics of Hawaii, I have had more than a lifetime dose of sun on my skin. My only armor was zinc oxide, which covered my nose almost continually. At night my body breathed the mentholated scent of Noxema which covered many a sunburn I also learned about the Aloe plant at an early age, and used its beach-side manner many times.

Vitamin D helps the body absorb calcium and phosphorus. **It is plentifully available in short sunshine basks, and it is available in fish liver oils and in fortified milk.**

REFLEX POINTS TO SUPPLEMENT HEALTH

Follow the same thirty second, three times per point technique you learned in the Facial Massage section.

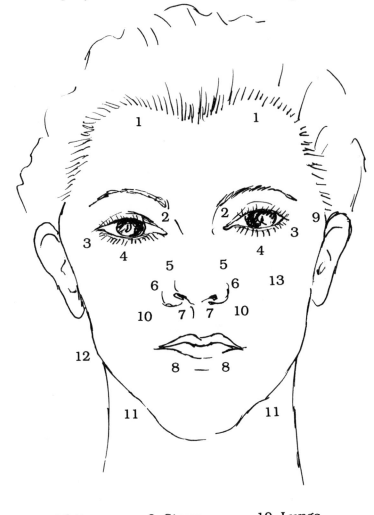

1. Mental fatigue
2. Headache
3. Digestion
4. Kidney
5. Intestine

6. Sinus
7. Spleen
8. Bladder
9. Thyroid

10. Lungs
11. Sex organs
12. Liver
13. Stomach

SUN, STRESS
AND SKIN AGING

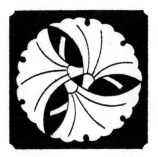

As skin ages, it tends to manufacture fewer new cells. Damaged cells are repaired at a slower and less efficient rate as well. The cell layers themselves become thinner and more brittle, resulting in a less protective and drier skin. The minute blood vessels begin to collapse and decrease in their efficiency, affecting sensation and the ability to clear waste particles from these layers. The most obvious of these ageing factors are wrinkling and sagging skin.

The thinning of the skin layers changes the fat distribution of the skin. Fat is redistributed to the thighs in women and to the waist in men. A balanced diet to keep the basal metabolism from slowing too much, and a good exercise program to ward off great accumulations in these areas are the best approach to working with this natural tendency.

The skin experiences two different types of ageing processes, namely chronological ageing and photoageing. The first is no more than our genetic disposition, the inherited tendency to age. I have always felt somewhat short-changed in the skin department, having very thin English/Irish/Scotch type skin. The layers are simply thinner than most other genetic types and more prone to suffer from internal and environmental stresses. I have learned though, that when this genetic skin type is at its healthiest, it of the most porcelain like, luminous looking skin in the world. All things have a positive side.

Photoageing has to do with sun exposure and its resulting damage. It is becoming more widely accepted among Dermatologists that photoaging is more of a threat to healthy skin than the natural ageing process.

The ultraviolet rays are absorbed into the epidermis, speeding up the production of melanin, which results in a tan. A tan is the body's natural defense system to protect the dermis layer, as the melanin absorbs some of the damaging ultraviolet rays. The average life of a tanning session is 7 to 25 days at the most. If tanning is overdone and peeling results, the peeling process takes as long to heal as the tan lasts.

Within the dermis layer is a large amount of collagen protein. When ultraviolet rays penetrate the dermis layer, the collagen fibers begin to break down. Because the collagen fibers give the skin its elasticity, a breakdown of these fibers results in a loss of the skins ability to stretch. The skin cells, when hardened by oxidation, collapse, resulting in a sagging and wrinkling of the skin, which then takes on a leathery appearance.

It is estimated that 3 out of 10 Americans will have some form of skin cancer during their lifetime. Further, 90% of skin cancers are caused from excessive sun exposure. Excessive sun exposure is not only cumulative, it is an irreversible kind of skin damage. The effects accumulate in the skin, breaking down the collagen and elastin proteins. Skin discolorations, "liver" spots and broken blood vessels are a result of accumulated sun damage.

There are certain dietary recommendations in working with cancers of any sort. With skin cancer in particular, the diet must be high in fresh fruits and vegetables, grains, azuki and mung beans, seaweeds, mushrooms, garlic, carrots, pumpkin, walnuts, dandelion greens, burdock root, asparagus, and licorice root. It is important to avoid meat, coffee, dairy products, spicy foods, high fat foods, stress, constipation and smoking. The best supplements are Vitamin A and E and Selenium.

Ones ethnic background has a lot to do with sun damage to skin. There are three basic categories of ethnic lines. Celtic, Scandinavian and Northern European people fit into the most susceptible to sun damage category. The people of Mediterranean descent comprise a somewhat less susceptible category. Hispanics and Asians have a general skin type that seldom burns. Africans fit into this third category or in some cases constitute a separate category because there are some Africans who simply are not skin sensitive to sun effects.

Other results of sun damaging are no less disturbing. Up to 90% of the skin's ageing results from ultraviolet light from sunshine as well as from interior lighting. Excessive ultraviolet light damages the genetic material within the cells, suppressing the skin's production of growth factors. Growth factors are known to stimulate immunity in the body, so a reduction of them means a less healthy immune system.

To minimize accumulated sun damage, first know your specific skin type. Additionally, make intelligent decisions about clothing, sunglass quality, sunblocks and sunscreens, and of course, the time of day you choose to expose your body to the sun.

I generally recommend the same advice to everyone I give facials and skin treatments. Avoid tanning and prolonged sun exposure during the mid-day hours of 10 A.M. to 3 P.M. Always use a sunscreen with appropriate coverage (I recommend a SPF 15 for face, hands, chest, and upper back, the most exposed areas of the body) and choose sunscreens wisely. There are some sunscreens that are actually detrimental to the skin because of their ingredients.

It may be of interest to note that during the 60's and early 70's an extremely intense period of sun spot activity increased the amount of ultraviolet rays in our atmosphere. The result is becoming evident in the number of skin cancer cases we are seeing today. We are experiencing the same increase in sun spot activity now, with an even more depleted ozone layer. The radiation we receive from the sun is extremely powerful and really needs to be taken in small doses!

STRESS

We are learning more and more ways to deal with stress as we learn more about its far reaching effects. One of the more recent findings is how stress affects the skin through the immune system. Each layer of the skin contains tiny Langerhans cells that direct blood cells to destroy invading bacteria and viruses. These blood cells, the T and B cells are also responsible for destroying cancer cells as they form in the body. Some of these T and B cells are produced in the blood for the skin alone. After they are formed, they migrate to the body's surface where they kill viruses and bacteria as they enter the pores of the skin. Here they confront little youth robbers called free radicals.

Free radicals are molecules created when the body uses oxygen. They are needed for many life functions including energy production, muscular contractions, oxygen absorption and hormone synthesis. Once their role in these functions is completed, they become molecular cast-offs no longer needed by the body.

Free radicals are unpaired electrons searching for an electron to attach to and become balanced. They attach themselves to cell walls, weakening and then destroying the cells. An excess of free radical activity destroys more cells than the body can create. The body becomes more stressed trying to deal with this devious activity, creating a vicious cycle that results in immunity impairment and tissue destruction. This tissue damage is most obvious in the skin and is one of the main causes of premature ageing.

Premature ageing and indeed, many diseases begin by the free radicals turning the body's lipids (fats) rancid. This is called lipid peroxidation. Our cells are surrounded by these lipids which make up the cell membrane. This oxidation by the free radicals causes the cell membrane to harden so that no nutrients can be absorbed into the cell. The skin cells, when hardened by oxidation, collapse, resulting in a sagging and wrinkling of the skin, which then takes on a leathery appearance. Once robbed of life sustaining nutrients, the cell dies, destroying tissue as a result.

Fortunately, the body's cells also produce antioxidant enzymes to counter the effect of free radical damage. However, with increased stresses to the body and mind, the antioxidant reserves in the body must likewise be increased. Lowering the stress factors, whether they be internal or external, such as pollution, radiation, poor nutrition, or overexertion is essential. Antioxidants which can penetrate the skin layers serve as receptors for the free radicals to attach to.

Antioxidants for skin application are vitamins. The molecules in vitamins A, C, and E are small enough to be absorbed into the skin and go to work on the underlying tissues. As many as 50 free radicals attach to each vitamin molecule before they are rejected from the body as toxic waste.

While the body rests at night, the skin is busy replacing damaged tissue and forming new cells. This is an ideal time to apply a moisturizer rich in antioxidant vitamins. Protecting the cells as they are forming is about as close as you can get to preventing cell oxidation.

Antioxidants may also be taken internally, as vitamins and as enzymes, to correct the damage from within. The main antioxidant enzyme is Superoxide dimutase, or SOD. It works together with another enzyme called catalase, both of which are naturally produced in the body. In fact, nearly 5,000,000 units of these enzymes are manufactured daily within the body.

Another major protector is the enzyme glutathione peroxidase which is the amino acid glutathione and the trace mineral selenium. Glutathione peroxidase is used primarily for skin related problems including wrinkling, dermatitis, eczema and skin cancer, but it also has a beneficial effect on allergies, liver disease, heart disease and chemical poisoning.

CREATIVE VISUALIZATION FOR THE SKIN

The connection between the mind and body has been one of the more important rediscoveries in modern medicine. Wholistic medicine has reintroduced the interconnectedness of mind, body and emotions, a concept that was understood and written about by our medical forefathers. Today, relaxation exercises and other stress-reduction techniques are prescribed by even conservative physicians.

It is near nearly impossible to separate the emotions from the skin's overall condition. The skin is closely connected with the nervous system. One square inch of skin contains thousands of nerve endings and receptors for perception of heat, cold, and other tactile sensations. The skin responds to emotional difficulties in many different ways, from minor itching to hives, warts, flare-ups, coloration and texture, and even skin tone. Understanding your emotions is one key to understanding your skin condition.

How does the skin respond to your mental and emotional state? Stress often induces the fight or flight syndrome, increasing the amount of adrenaline in the bloodstream. The endocrine glands release hormones which increase respiration, heartbeat, blood sugar and perspiration. The lymph and digestive system are slowed down, resulting in a decrease of toxic waste removal from the body. These toxins build up in the body and are diverted to the liver and the skin. The blood flow to the skin is then slowed down, decreasing moisture and vital skin nutrients to the skin tissues. The result is drier skin.

True beauty is more than skin deep. It is an expression of how we feel about ourselves. The result of cosmetic applications of Aromatherapy are also far from skin deep; a scent such as rose, while being calming and soothing to mature or sensitive skin is also responsible for easing insomnia and depression.

According to the well known biochemist Marguerite Maury, who has done a great deal of research into Aromatherapy, fragrances have a profound effect on the psychic and mental states of a person. Her research showed that the power of perception becomes clearer and more acute with Aromatherapy applications.

By creating certain images in your mind, you can determine, to a degree, a healthier skin. Imagining ideal conditions and situations that will make your skin feel better helps to temporarily relieve the symptoms your skin may be experiencing. You are setting up an internal climate that is more receptive to a healthier skin. Such slight physiological changes have been demonstrated to have positive results in the thousands of people who practice positive imagery.

Before beginning your initial imagery exercise, write down the things that you know make your skin feel better and then the things that make it feel worse. Include places, times, and let your imagination create your ideal environment (is there anything here that you can actually implement in your home to improve the conditions?) with as much detail and as clearly as you can.

If you love fine scented creams, imagine yourself enveloped in a fragrant pond of skin lotion made with the expressed oils of your favorite flowers. Your pores are little mouths drinking in this delicious nectar. Multiply the feeling of satiation and pleasure. Your skin will respond favorably as your mind eases into the enjoyment of your private paradise.

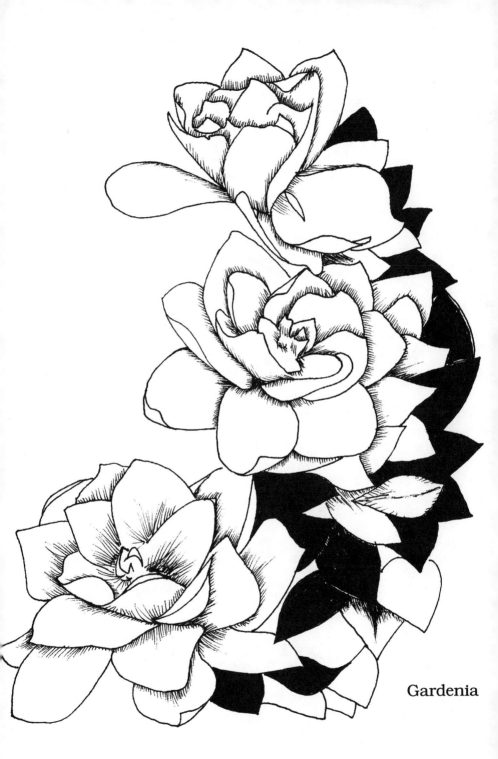

Gardenia

PART III

THE AT HOME SPA

Fair is the bird on lustrous wings
And stars through all nights silent hours;
But first, of all created things,
In wondrous beauty stand the flowers.

From Indigenous Flowers of the Hawaiian Islands
by Mrs. Francis Sinclair

ADORNMENT
AROMATHERAPY

To many a person, make-up is a face of acceptance, a conformity to a greater-than-self image, a collective face, a cultural coloration. The art of making up a face is as individualized as an art can be, each face a unique palate to adorn with color. A simple knowledge of color, one's skin tone, and an understanding of one's own facial composition are the skills required. One is either yellow toned (warm colors) or blue toned (cool colors). This is determined by looking at the skin and blood veins at the inside fold of the elbow.

Makeup is for me a delightful way to play with and celebrate my self image. I use makeup to correctively color my face as well, shading a nose I often deem too large, defining cheekbones that hardly show through my chipmunk cheeks, and transforming my thin English upper lip into a semblance of a Cupids' bow, a relaxed one at that.

To achieve a finished and soft coloration, a good set of brushes is helpful. You will want a lip brush, a blunt blush brush, a full soft brush for loose powder, an eyelid brush and an eyebrow brush (an old toothbrush will do). Keep these brushes clean by washing with a mild soap and warm water.

I prefer makeup that is simple, fresh, easy to use, and appealing. Of the many formulas I have made over the years, these are among my favorites:

Rosebud Lips

1/2 cup vegetable oil (Olive, Sweet Almond,
 Sesame, Wheat germ)
1/2 cup red Rose petals
1 Tbs. Vitamin E oil
1 Tbs. Honey
1 oz. Beeswax

Blend fresh rose petals with the oil, strain. Heat all ingredients together until beeswax has melted. Add 6 drops Moroccan or Bulgarian Rose oil, pour into small, clean, recycled containers, and share with friends. Us a lip brush for a long lasting application.

Beet Cheeks

To the same formula, add 1-2 teaspoons of dried beet powder. This will make a natural glow of pink tint. For a darker color, add 1/2 teaspoon of Indian Earth or a natural mineral color. The Rose essential oil lends a bit of color to the formulas as well.

Face Powder

A face powder will absorb excess moisture, even the skin tone, and lend a soft look to the skin. Simply combine a little Cornstarch and/or Rice flour with some Cinnamon powder to the shade desired. The Cinnamon will lightly fragrance the powder. Add a bit of powdered Beet for a rosy glow, or a bit of crushed pearls for a delicate translucence. You can experiment with the dried powdered flowers of Nasturtium, Calendula, Rose, Hibiscus, or Blue Malva, and Beets for shades varying from peach to plum.

Midnight Eyes

This is really an ancient Egyptian formula for the eyelids. I have added one ingredient which I feel lends a soft smoky look. Simply grind a few tablespoons of wood ashes (someone you know has a woodstove, I hope) to a fine powder with a mortar and pestle. Add a pinch or more of Spirulina powder to give a hint of green. A pinch of Blue Malva flower powder will provide a violet hue. A pinch made into a thin paste with a drop of water may be applied as an eyeliner as well. Keep the powder blend in a clean, airtight container.

THE AROMATIC BODY

It is certainly easy to simply pick products from the skin care section of your salon or health food store, and create an instant skin care center at home. It is far more time consuming to grow, gather, combine, and bottle such products yourself. However, the rewards of such labors are many. Not only will you be acquiring an understanding of the essences of flowers and plant materials, their sensual and therapeutic potencies, but you will also be able to learn which ingredients are best suited for your personal skin type by formulating for yourself.

I have collected formulas from my own practice and personal experimentation. They are meant as a springboard for you to delve into the heart of the flower, its precious gifts to be the base of your healing potions and unguents. Allow these flower exudations to work their magic in creating greater balance and unity between the skin, mind and emotions.

Wherever I have left the Essential Oil choice open, I intend for you to choose oils that pertain to your own skin type. All of the formulas are designed for both men and women as well as their children.

Morning Elixir
or Instant Aromatherapy

Stroll through a flower garden before the flower dew has evaporated. Upon greeting a fragrant bloom, sip the dew from the petals.

Best to avoid sipping from flowers along roadsides where plants may be sprayed or dusty. Investigate the wild flowers you may have around you.

In Hawaii I am privy to the exotic exudations of Tuberose, Jasmine, Honeysuckle, Gardenia, Rose. Each time I drink of a flowers' essence, I feel invited by Nature to enjoy the most delicate of her gifts.

91

RECIPES FOR REJUVENATION

Skin Tonic

Cosmetologists have long held that the skin is better cleansed and refreshed by the use of a vinegar wash. Vinegar washes have been used in skin care for centuries, and not only are they very inexpensive and easy to make, they provide an important aid by keeping the skin's PH slightly acidic. This protection of the acid mantel keeps bacteria in check and helps the skin to maintain a healthy state. This very basic cosmetic is beneficial to all skin types.

> 1/4 oz. Apple Cider Vinegar
> 7 3/4 oz. Water
> 15 drops Essential Oil

Combine 3 ingredients. Pour into spray bottle, spritz face and body to cool and refresh skin throughout the day. Makes 8 ounces. Shake before each use.

Witch Hazel Skin Toner

1/2 cup Witch Hazel
2 teaspoons Vegetable Glycerin
2 Tbs. Aloe Vera Juice
5 drops desired essential oil, according to skin
    type

Combine all ingredients. Shake well before each use. Use in a mister during the day for extra hydration or saturate a cotton pad to apply after cleansing. Very gentle and soothing to all skin types. Makes 5 ounces.

Skin Polish

This is such an easy and inexpensive formula for removing dead skin cell buildup over the body. It has been used for centuries as a natural exfoliant. The buildup of dead skin cells gives the skin a ruddy, dull appearance, and a simple rubbing with this paste leaves the skin looking more vibrant and aglow with health.

1/4 cup Cornmeal
1/4 cup Oats, ground
2 Tbs. Orris Root powder (optional)

Combine ingredients. Store in closed container. Mix 1 Tbs. with enough water to make a thick paste in palm of hand. Rub over face in small circular motions, paying particular attention to clogged pore and blackhead areas. Rinse with lukewarm water. Follow with a toner and moisturizer.

Daily Skin Brushing

Body brushing is a very old skin care practice. It improves circulation and helps the lymph to move toxins from the body.

Dry brush massage stimulates nerve endings, invigorates the nervous system, helps move fat cells and break up cellulite, increases muscle tone and improves immune system functions. A daily five minute body brushing will make your skin and body feel more alert and awake.

This simple technique is best done with a vegetable bristle brush. One with a long handle will help to cover the back side of the body more easily. You may want to rub 3-5 drops of a chosen essential oil over the bristles to increase the effectiveness of the routine. Use light upward strokes from the soles of the feet to the heart and from the palms of the hand in toward the heart. Use long sweeping strokes with a light pressure. A good way to stimulate lymphatic circulation is to rotate the brush back and forth under the armpits. Follow brushing with a warm bath or shower.

Lavender Cleansing Cream

1 egg yolk
1/2 cup Vegetable Oil
1 teaspoon Borax
1 cup hot water
2 Tbs. Witch Hazel
7 drops Lavender Oil

Heat vegetable oil (I prefer sweet almond or avocado oil) to 100 degrees or until hot to the touch. Do the same with the water, borax, and witch hazel in a separate small pan. You may use a microwave for this. Put oil in a blender. Add the egg yolk. Press stir button. Slowly add the hot water blend in a thin stream. Blend for a few minutes while adding the essential oil.

Pour a week's amount into a small jar. Store the rest of your cleanser in the refrigerator. Use instead of soap to remove make-up or to cleanse face. Wipe cleanser off with a warm washcloth or cotton saturated with SKIN TONIC.

Rose Oat Cleansing Milk

It has long been known that oats are cleansing and nourishing to the skin. This formula takes advantage of these properties, plus the skin softening benefits of glycerin and Rose oil. This is an ideal formula for all skin types.

    1/4 cup Oats
    1 cup hot water
    2 Tbs. Glycerin
    2 Tbs. Liquid soap
    5 drops Rose oil

Soak oats in water, blend. Make sure the blender liquefies the oats. Combine ingredients. Blend with Oat mixture. Store in cool place. Massage 1 Tbs. into face. Wipe off with warm wash cloth or cotton saturated with Skin Tonic or Witch Hazel Skin Toner. Makes 1 1/2 cups.

Pore Cleansing Lotion

To soften and help emulsify unwanted debris in the pores, a disencrustant is applied after cleansing and before extractions or a mask. A very simple formula is to mix 1 Tbs. Baking Soda with 1 pint water. Add 5 drops of Thyme or Rosemary oil. Store in a closed container. Shake well before applying. Saturate cotton and moisten skin. The baking soda breaks the emulsion of the clogging oils, making it easier to remove the trapped debris. The mask will further help by lifting the oils to the surface. If the pore needs some extraction by hand, follow the directions for extractions in the facial.

Herbal Shaving Cream

2 ounces old soap ends
2 ounces water
1 teaspoon Borax
1 Tbs. Vegetable Glycerin
2 drops Sage Oil
2 drops Thyme Oil
2 drops Lavender Oil

In a small pan, melt soap chips and borax in the water over low heat. Stir in other ingredients. Pour into shaving cup, let cool and harden. Use with a shaving brush for a skin soothing shave and a light fresh scent. Good for all skin types, on legs, underarms, and beards.

Lavender Rose Lotion

1 1/2 cups water
1 cup Sweet Almond Oil
1/2 ounce beeswax
10 drops Lavender oil
5 drops Rose Geranium, Bulgarian Rose or
    Moroccan Rose Oil

Melt beeswax in oil over low heat. Heat water separately. Slowly add water in a steady stream while beating oil mixture with electric mixer or a wisk. Add essential oils, blending on low. Pour into small, clean bottles. Refrigerate excess. My favorite all purpose skin cream, effective on all skin types.

Masks

Clays are a very good ingredient in masks because they are stimulating, toning, and cleansing to all skin types. Clay is rich in minerals such as Silica, Magnesium oxide, Iron oxide and Calcium oxide. Certain clays are more stimulating than others, with varying degrees of balancing capabilities. Most drug stores sell clay in the form of Kaolin. Health food stores carry the more varieties of clays, rose clay being my favorite.

Green clay- good for oily skin.
White clay- good for delicate skin.
Rose clay-good for normal to oily skin.
Blue clay- good for sensitive, dry skin.

Quick Clay Mask

To make a quick mask for normal to oily skin, combine 3 Tbs. of any clay with 3 drops essential oil (Lavender, Rose and Geranium are wonderful) and enough hot water to make a thin paste. Brush on face, rest for 10 minutes, rinse off with warm, then cool water.

To make a quick mask for dry and sensitive skin, mix 3 Tbs. white clay with 1 Tbs. yogurt and 3 drops essential oil of Chamomile, Neroli or Rose. Follow same procedure.

Avocado Mask
For Dry and Mature Skin

1/2 Avocado
1 Tbs. Yogurt, unflavored
3 drops Chamomile oil
1 Tbs. Brewers yeast

This mask is rich in vitamin E to nourish and revive tired, dry skin. Blend Avocado with yogurt until fluffy. Scrape into small bowl. Stir in oil. Pat or brush over face, rest for 20 minutes. Rinse with warm, then cool water. Makes 1 treatment. This mask should be made fresh each time, and excess should be stored in refrigerator for no more than 3 days.

Gel Mask

A gel based mask is ideal for dry skin types or for frequent mask applications. They store well in the refrigerator, and can be used over the entire body for a skin softening treatment.

3 oz. water
3 oz. Vegetable Glycerin
1 Tbs. Agar (seaweed powder)

Stir glycerin and agar over heat until agar is incorporated. Add water, let stand overnight to thicken. This is about 10 facial applications worth of base. Add 3 drops essential oils per facial application.

Ingredients I like to add to this base are fresh papaya, honey, avocado, vitamins A and E, strong Herbal teas.

For a cooling and soothing treat to tired feet and legs, mix 3-5 drops Peppermint oil with Gel Mask. The stimulating action of Peppermint affects the nerve endings in a mildly invigorating way, easing tension and soreness.

Skin To Skin Mask

Living in the islands I have the pleasure of tree ripened papayas. My favorite breakfast treat is to sit in the early morning sun with a papaya half into which I put a tablespoon of unroasted sesame butter. After spooning out the papaya fruit, I rub the inside of the skin over my face and neck, pressing the remaining juices into my skin. I rest in the sun for 10 minutes, feeling the warmth, smelling the fruit, and softening my skin with the enzymatic action of the papain in the papaya. A quick dip in the ocean removes the pulp and leaves my skin feeling more awake and looking softer.

Mermaids/Mermen Mask

1 cup clay
1 cup Powdered Kelp
1/2 cup Spirulina powder
10 drops per treatment Essential oils

Mix and store in tight container. Use essential oils according to skin type.

For a facial, mix 2 Tbs. powder with enough hot water to make a thick paste. Brush or pat onto clean, towel warmed face, rest for 15-20 minutes. Use 5 drops essential oil for each face mask.

For a body mask, mix three handfuls of powder with enough hot water to make a paste thin enough to spread over the body. Rub quickly over just bathed body, wrap in hot, damp sheet, cover with blankets, and rest for 20 minutes.

For a bath, add 1/2 cup (or more, if desired) to the bath, with 10 drops essential oils. Relax in bath for 20 minutes. This may be done before the body mask.

INSTANT SEAWEED MASK

2 sheets Nori (seaweed sheets for sushi rolls)
2 drops Neroli Oil (optional)

Warm a clean face with hot, moist towel. Mix Neroli with 1 teaspoon of very light oil (i.e. Apricot Kernel) and apply to face and neck. Run Nori sheets under warm water but do not soak them. Apply each sheet to one half of the face, leaving an opening for the nose. Leave on for 20 minutes, peel off Nori, and mist face with a toner or vinegar wash. The Neroli oil, a member of the Orange family, is a skin cell regenerator and with the remineralizing properties of the seaweed, the treatment is simple and effective.

Thalassotherapy is the use of sea water and sea plants to promote health and beauty. The theory is that the chemical composition of sea water is within 2% identical to human plasma. Seaweeds have a remarkable softening, remineralizing, moisturizing and firming effect on the skin. They contain all of the building blocks of life: minerals, trace elements, amino acids, vitamins, and other nutrients.

Seaweeds help to detoxify tissues and regulate blood circulation in the body. The high iodine content stimulates the thyroid gland. This increases the metabolic action and the circulation, speeding up the detoxification process of the body. This action helps to decrease cellulite deposits.

A primordial pleasure is found in seaweed body treatments. The warm seaweed smell enrobes the body in Neptunian nutrients. Combined with Aromatherapy, it is a powerfully nourishing and cleansing treatment of the skin and its underlying functions. The hydrating qualities of the seaweeds combined with the drawing power of a clay, and balancing power of the essential oils will offer a revitalizing treatment.

There are thousands of types of seaweed. Most commonly used in skin care preparations are Laminaria, Fucus Vesiculosus (Kelp), and Ascophylium.

Facial Massage Oils

Dry/Sensitive Skin:
3 oz. Apricot Kernel oil
3 drops Rose oil
3 drops Lavender oil
3 drops Myrrh oil
3 drops Chamomile oil

Mature Skin:
3 oz. Apricot Kernel oil
1 Tbs. Vitamin E oil
5 drops Rose oil
5 drops Jasmine oil
5 drops Neroli oil

Normal/Combination Skin:
3 oz. Sweet Almond oil
3 drops Lavender oil
3 drops Geranium oil
3 drops Ylang Ylang oil
3 drops Orange oil

Oily/Acne Skin:
2 oz. Glycerin
1 oz. Water
3 drops Rosemary oil
3 drops Cedar oil
3 drops Sandalwood oil

Bath Gel

This is a favorite bath treat. Its rich velvet texture leaves a satiny smooth shine on the skin. The herbs are both skin softening and mentally calming.

> 1 egg yolk
> 1/4 cup Sesame or Almond oil
> 2 cups Water
> 10 drops Lavender
> 10 drops Sage
> 10 drops Verbena

Blend oil and egg yolk. Slowly add water in a thin stream. Stir in essential oils. Store in refrigerator. Use 1/4 cup per bath.

Aphrodite's Bath Oil

> 1 cup Olive oil
> 10 drops Sandalwood oil
> 10 drops Clove oil
> 10 drops Cedarwood oil
> 10 drops Citrus oil (Lemon, Orange, Bergamot)

Combine all ingredients. Pour 2 Tbs. into bath just before getting in. Rest in bath for 15 minutes. Gently pat skin dry or air dry body. This is especially good for dry, tired skin. The blend is delightfully calming, one I first experienced on Crete, near the ruins of Knossos, where elaborate aqueducts were built for bathing pleasures.

Cleopatra's Bath

1 cup instant Powdered Milk
1 cup Epsom Salts
10 drops Orange oil
10 drops Ylang Ylang oil

Combine all ingredients, store in closed container. Makes 3 baths. A skin soothing and softening treatment. It is known that Cleopatra's beauty regime included milk baths. The Epsom salts were probably not used by Cleopatra though I have added them because of their drawing and mineralizing benefits. Epsom salts relieve muscle strain as they help to pull toxins from the skin tissues.

Aromatic Bath Salts

1 cup Borax
3 cup Epsom Salts
10 drops Eucalyptus oil
10 drops Pine or Birch oil
10 drops Thyme oil

Combine all ingredients and shake well. Store in closed container. Use one to two cups per bath. Soak for 20 minutes.

Deodorants and Body Powders

Many commercial deodorants contain aluminum chlorohydrate, a toxic substance suspected in Alzheimer development, cancer, ulcers, and heart disease. Prolonged daily use of such deodorants tax the lymph system, of which the main glands are in the armpits. A weakened lymph system weakens the immune system, resulting in a less healthy state of being.

Deodorant Spray

10 drops Lavender
5 drops Thyme
5 drops Sage
10 drops Calendula
1/2 cup Water
2 Tbs. Alcohol

Combine oils with alcohol, add water. Pour into pump spray bottle. Shake before use. The oils can also be stirred into 1/2 cup cornstarch for a powder deodorant.

Tropic Tradewinds Body Powder

1 cup Cornstarch
2 Tbs. Baking soda
10 drops Jasmine oil
5 drops Orange oil

Combine powders, stir in oils. Store in 1 cup size container. Dust over body with large powder brush or puff. The baking soda helps to absorb and neutralize body odors. The Jasmine and Orange oils combine to create a tantalizing and skin revitalizing treatment beneficial in all climates.

Purifying Body Powder

1 cup Cornstarch
1 cup Rice flour
10 drops Sandalwood oil
10 drops Cedar oil
5 drops Vetiver oil

Combine powders, stir in oils. Store in a 2 cup size container with tight fitting lid. Wonderful outdoors scent and a great deodorant powder, foot powder, and all over body powder. This is especially nice on dry or sensitive skin. It is a most attractive scent on men.

Rose Moisturizing Powder

1 cup Cornstarch
1 cup Rose clay
10 drops Rose Oil
1 Tbs. Olive oil

Drizzle Olive oil over ingredients and shake well. This is especially good for babies and for extremely dry and sensitive skin.

Perfumes

The word perfume derives from the ancient practice of burning scented materials for religious and ceremonial purposes; per (through) fumun (smoke). I am including these formulas because they are my favorite of the basic classic blends. You may want to personalize blends for your own skin type or for particular mood enhancement. I recommend using a pure grain alcohol available in liquor stores as Everclear alcohol, 90 proof. To each of the below formulas, add 1 ounce Alcohol. Store perfumes in tightly stoppered bottles or atomizers. To perfume the home, rub a few drops over the lamp bulbs before turning them on at night. The heat of the bulb will diffuse the scent throughout the room.

Peacefully

A soothing fresh scent for both men and women. May add 4 ounces of Witch Hazel to make a refreshing skin splash.

100 drops Orange oil
75 drops Lemon oil
50 drops Bergamot oil
25 drops Geranium oil
20 drops Storax or Benzoin

Elysium

A lively breeze of scent that the whole family loves. An ideal after-shave for men and women.

100 drops Lemon oil
100 drops Thyme oil
50 drops Sage oil
5 drops Rosemary oil
1 ounce Alcohol
6 ounces Witch Hazel

Dilute oils in Alcohol. Add Witch Hazel. Shake before each use.

Ariel At Play

A light, classic blend

50 drops Orange oil
15 drops Neroli
15 drops Rose
5 drops Jasmine
2 drops Benzoin

Dream Divine

A musky blend to set a mood of love

100 drops Bergamot oil
40 drops Sandalwood oil
20 drops Patchouli oil
10 drops Storax or Labdanum oil
10 drops Lavender
5 drops Rose

Say Yes

A quiet, unassuming blend that invites a deep relaxation response. It wears well on women and men.

60 drops Lavender oil
10 drops Neroli oil
5 drops Rosemary oil

Making Your Own Flower Essence

Here are two very simple ways to retrieve the essence and healing properties from flowers or herbs.

Sunshine Method

Fill a glass, stainless, or ceramic bowl with rain, spring or distilled water. Take the bowl to the flower source, and begin pinching the flowers from their stems, placing them directly in the water. When the water surface is completely covered with flowers, place the bowl in the direct sun where no shadows will pass over it. You want full sunlight to most effectively distill the essences. At the end of the day, strain the flowers (you may want to use a few in your evening salad or as a garnish), pour the water into a clean bottle, and preserve in the refrigerator. Use this potent flower extraction by the droplet in masks, toners, facial steams, cleansers, and creams. Put a few drops into a glass of water for an aromatic elixir and float a flower in the glass.

You may want to collect the thin film of essential oil that floats to the surface of the bowl. Take a Q-Tip or small piece of cotton and skim the surface of the water, pressing the drops into a small clean bottle. Add some grain alcohol to this collection of oils, and use as an essential oil.

Boiling Method

Gather flowers in the morning and put into saucepan, covering with water. Bring to a light boil, and simmer, uncovered, for 1/2 hour. Cool, remove the flowers, strain into a clean bottle. Store and use as above.

MORE FUN THINGS TO DO WITH ESSENTIAL OILS

1. Two drops Orange, Lemon, Thyme or Sage oil on an herbal tea bag. Steep in 1 cup hot water. Divine yourself with a cup of tea.

2. A few drops on a light bulb before lighting a room.

3. A few drops to fine laundry or machine wash.

4. A few drops on a cotton ball, placed in drawers and cupboards, shoes, suitcases, anything stored.

5. A few drops to the vacuum cleaner filter.

6. A few drops on hot pads; the heat from the stove on the pot holder will scent the whole kitchen.

7. A few drops on a handkerchief is instant Aromatherapy.

8. 10 drops in 1/2 quart hot water. Immerse washcloth and apply damp cloth to any part of the body for specific treatment.

9. 5 drops Lavender, Sage or Peppermint oil in 3 tablespoons of honey. Take 1 teaspoon.

10. 10 -20 drops into hot tub. Get into tub while adding oils for full vaporizing effect.

ALEXANDRA'S
ESSENTIAL APOTHECARY

Angelica: An earthy scent of roots gives a balancing effect to this aphrodisiac oil. It is very toning to the reproductive system and stimulating to the glandular system. It is used in Chinese medicine to relieve headaches. I feel it sharpens my concentration and overall vitality, and use a few drops of it in all of my personal blends.

Geranium: A skin strengthening oil, stimulating to the circulation and adrenal glands, increases the body's vital energy. I often use it in a vaporizer or rub it on a candle to scent the room where I work.

Basil: One of the best stimulant oils for mental clarity. A little bottle is kept at my writing table as a coffee alternative. I often end my facials with a misting of Basil water to 'wake up' the client.

Lavender: Always with me, Lavender is calming, soothing and regenerating to the skin. It relaxes the mind and calms the spirit. I keep a sachet of lavender flowers in my car and can be seen taking frequent sniffs in traffic jams!

Neroli: There is a hypnotic quality to Neroli that completely tantalizes me. It has been the prime oil in my night face blend for years, and I believe it has been chiefly responsible for balancing my dry skin condition.

Lemon: Most of my facials include Lemon oil because it stimulates the function of the epidermis. It oxygenates purifies the tissues. The skin feels toned, firmed and refreshed. It stimulates the development of red blood cells, increasing the body's immunity. I also use it in baths, combined with Neroli, for a most rejuvenating effect on my senses and skin.

Vetiver: A most penetrating oil, working on the deepest layers of the skin. It stimulates the blood, increasing the cleansing and strengthening action of the connective tissues. I use a couple of drops in every facial massage blend. It works wonderfully with Sandalwood oil.

Oak Moss: When I first discovered Oak Moss, my senses were overwhelmed. I felt the centuries of use of this forest plant all in an instant, and immediately chose it as my companion herb. Oak Moss is supremely soothing and nourishing to the skin and senses. The oil is rich and redolent like being buried in forest mosses. I use it mixed with vegetable oils for a body lotion. Oak Moss may also be sold as Tree Moss, and is bright green in color.

Gardenia: I suppose Gardenias are to an island girl what Magnolias are to a southern girl, the essence of purity married with a sweet sensuality. Pleasant thoughts are born in the whiff of a Gardenia. Over the years that I have been extracting the oil on the slopes of Mauna Kea, I have become convinced that this flower aids in connecting the body, mind, and spirit. Try floating a Gardenia blossom in a brandy snifter half filled with water, and placing it where you will be able to breathe in its wafting magic.

Jasmine: I love Jasmine for its gentle treatment to the skin and its subtle, arousing touch to the senses. I also enjoy using a drop in my facial steam so I can breathe it in for a while.

RECOMMENDED READING

Anderson, Bruce, Ecologue: The Environmental Catalogue
    and Consumer's Guide for a Safe Earth.
    A necessary resource book for every consumer.

Being Beautiful: Deciding for Yourself.
    Send $10.00 to Center for the Study of Responsive
    Law, P.O. Box 19367, Washington D.C. 20036.
    Selected readings with an introduction by Ralph
    Nader.

Caldicott, Helen, If You Love This Planet - A Plan To Heal
    The Earth, W.W. Norton.

Commoner, Barry, Making Peace with the Planet.
    Pantheon Press.
    Awakening and empowering information.

Cuningham, Scott, Magical Aromatherapy.
    An entertaining and informative little book worth
    having in a collection.

Dadd, Debra Lynn, Nontoxic, Natural, & Earthwise.
    How you can take responsibility for your part on the
    planet.

Davis, Patricia, Aromatherapy from A to Z.
    Easy reference of a wide selection of plant essences.

Diamond, Denise, Living with the Flowers: A Guide to
    Bringing Flowers into your Daily Life. A delightfully
    written and illustrated invitation to experience your
    garden as you never have before. Lots of recipes
    lore, facts, and anecdotes about flowers.

Diamond, Irene and Gloria Orenstein, Reweaving the
    World. A collection of essays about the emergence of
    Ecofeminism, a fresh look at healing ourselves and
    our planet by reweaving poetic vision through the
    social, economic, and political structures of the
    world.

Hasselbring, Bobbi, Medical Self-Care Book of Women's
Health. Doubleday, 1988. Very informative about
safe cosmetics and healthful beauty practices.

Jackson, Judith, Scentual Touch.
Covers Aromatherapy body massage. Very well done.

Kenton, Leslie, The Joy of Beauty.
An excellent reference book.

Kushi, Mishio, Your Face Never Lies. Covers diagnosing
body health through 'reading' the face, with an
emphasis on diet. Valuable reference book.

Lavabe, Marcel, Handbook of Aromatherapy.
Student's practical on Aromatherapy.

Price, Shirley, Practical Aromatherapy.
Concise collection of essences and their properties.

Rose, Jeanne, Kitchen Cosmetics. Using herbs, fruits and
eatables in natural cosmetics. The Aromatherapy
Book. Comprehensive reading and good fun.

Thomas, Virginia Castleton, My Secrets of Natural Beauty.
Collection of good basic body care formulas.

Tisserand, Maggie, Aromatherapy for Women.
Compact information for women of all ages.

Tisserand, Robert, The Art of Aromatherapy.
Informative how-to of Aromatherapy.

Teagarden, Iona, Acupressure Way of Health:
Jin Shin Do. Simple acupressure approach to facial
toning and overall health.

Valnet, Jean, Practice of Aromatherapy.
A necessity on all Aromatherapist's shelves.

Winter, Ruth, A Dictionary of Cosmetic Ingredients: Complete Information About the Harmful and Desirable
Ingredients found in Men's and Women's Cosmetics.
A good reference book for the formulator and the
cosmetics   buyer.

Wolf, Naomi, The Beauty Myth: How Images Of Women
Are Used Against Women. Morrow, N.Y. A very
rousing exposure of our cultural obsession with
beauty.

MAIL ORDER
SOURCE DIRECTORY

Alexandra Avery, P.O. Box 231, Kailua, HI 96734. Facial
and skin care, plant perfumes, custom blending.

Aphrodesia, 282 Bleeker St. N.Y., N.Y. 10018. Essential
oils, formula supplies.

Aroma Vera, P.O. Box 3384 So. Robertson Pl. L.A., CA.
90034. Essential oils, skin care.

Aromatherapy Supplies, 52 St. Aubyn's Rd., Fishersgate,
Brighton, Sussex, England. Essential oils, books,
skin care.

Aura Cacia, P.O. Box 391, Weaverville, CA. Essential oils,
skin care.

Balancing Botanicals, P.O. Box 2514, Fair Oaks, CA
95628. A lovely collection of 6 skin soothing
Aromabalms.

Body Love, P.O. Box 7542, Santa Cruz, CA. 95061. Skin
care, essential oils and Goddess blends.

Elias, P.O. Box 313, Ojai, CA. 93023. Divine body oils and
aromatic waters for the skin and palate.

Essence Aromatherapy, 1760 W. 34 Ave. Eugene, OR
97405. Beautiful body oils, annoints, candles.

Geremy Rose, P.O. Box 1947, Brattleboro VT 05301. Skin
care.

Jeanne Rose New Age Creations, 219 Carl St. San Francisco, CA 94117. Skin Care, books, education program.

Judith Jackson, 96 Lewis St., Greenwich, CT 06830. Body oils, a practical book, The Scentual Touch.

Kathy Keville, 14648 Pear Tree Lane, Nevada City, CA 95959. Aromatherapy educator and author.

Leydet Oils, P.O. Box 2354, Fair Oaks, CA 95628. Essential oils, perfumes, books.

Liberty Oils, 8120 S.E. Stark, Portland, OR 97213. Essential oils, breath fresheners.

Lifetree Aromatrix, 3949 Longridge Ave., Sherman Oaks, CA. 91423. Essential oils, Aromatic consulting and Aromatherapy kit.

Nuzzi-St. Clair, Debra, 997 Dixon Rd. Boulder, CO 80302. Essential Oil inhalers, Herbal study video.

Original Swiss Aromatics, P.O. Box 606, San Rafael, CA. 94915. Essential oils, education program.

Santa Fe Fragrance, P.O. Box 282, Santa Fe, NM. 87504. Aromatic consulting, perfumes.

Simplers Botanical Company, P.O. Box 39, Forestville, CA 95436. Simple and pure Aromatherapy skin care.

Talisman, 68 Tinker St., Woodstock, N.Y. 12498. Essential oils, perfumes.

The Essential Oil Company, P.O. Box 206, Lake Oswego, OR. 97034. Essential oils, Aromatherapy Massage Video, Natural Healing Home Study Course.

Tiferet, 2555 Portland St. Eugene, OR. 97405. Essential oils, perfumes.

Tisserand Inst. 3 Shurley St. Hove, Easty Sussex, England 8N15NB, Essential oils, books, education program.

Weeds of Worth, 540 W. Main St. Northboro, MA 01532.
Body oils and salves.

Weleda, 841 Main P.O. Box 769, Spring Valley, N.Y.
10977. Quality skin care products.

Miscellaneous

Ageless Beauty Enzymes, Biotec Foods, One of the best
sources of anti-oxidants I've found. Call for information and nearest Health Food Store source to you.
1-800 468-7578, Hawaii.

Home Health Products, 32 page catalog of basic care for
health, beauty and wellness.
1-800 284- 9123, Ext. 202, Florida.

Lucas Steamer, described on page 50, for professional and
home use, $325. 42 Palione Place, Kailua, HI 96734.

Spirulina, For use in skin care, order powder not tablets.
Earthrise Co., P.O. Box 1196, San Rafael, CA 94915.
Pegasus Center, 1A Robbins Lane, Rocky Hill, CT
06067.
Microlight Nutritional Products, 124 Rhodesia Beach
Rd., Bay Center, WA 98527,1-800 338 2821.

Summer Rose, Anne Williams, Earthsong Productions,
P.O.Box 780, Sedona, Arizona, 86336. A journey into
the heart of the Rose.

Recycled Paper Products

Seventh Generation, 1-800 4561177, Vermont. From toilet
paper to biodegradable cleaners.

Green Cross paper products, (napkins, towels, tissues)
contain 100 percent recycled paper fibers and are
dioxin free. They are available in supermarkets.

BIBLIOGRAPHY

Bienfang. The Subtle Sense. Norman, Oklahoma. 1946.

Davis, Patricia. Aromatherapy, an A-Z, Daniel Pub., UK, 1988.

Fritsche Brothers. Perfumers Handbook and Catalog. N.Y. 1944.

Gumbel, Dietrich. Principles of Holistic Skin Therapy with Herbal Essences. Medicina Biologica. Portland, OR 97211.

Jessee, Jill. Perfume Album. Robert Krieger Publisher. N.Y. 1974.

Kennett, Frances. History of Perfume. Harrap, London. 1975.

Kenton, Leslie. The Joy of Beauty. Doubleday and Company. N.Y. 1983.

Lavabre, Marcel. The Handbook of Aromatherapy. USA, 1986.

LeGallienne, Richard. The Romance of Perfume. N.Y. 1928.

McKenzie, Dan, M.D. Aromatics and the Soul. London. 1923.

Naves, Dr. Y.R. and Mazuyer, G. Natural Perfume Materials. N.Y. 1947.

Novick, Nelson Lee, M.D. Super Skin. C.N. Potter, Inc. Publishers. N.Y. 1988.

Read, John. The Alchemist in Life. Literature, and Art. London. 1947.

Sagarin, Edward. The Science and Art of Perfumery. McGraw Hill, N.Y. 1945.

Thompson, C.J.S. The Mystery and Lure of Perfume. The Bodley Head Ltd., London. 1927.

Tisserand, Robert, The Art of Aromatherapy. New York. 1977.

Valnet, Dr. Jean. Aromatherapy. New York. 1980.

ESSENTIAL LIVING

There is more . . . beyond the pleasures of treating the skin and senses with aromas and other gifts of the plant kingdom, there is the journey inward, toward an essential expression of self.

We are all co-creators with unique, individual expressions. Choosing to work from our personal essence is key to living a meaningful life. We all have the power to change our lives, and in doing so, to play a part in changing the world. We are co-creating a world of peaceful, healthy living. We are co-creating with nature, restoring the Earth and humankind as well.

Start with what helps you to love yourself fully. Affirming your personal potential and believing you are a part of the whole picture of evolution is essential to understanding planetary potential. We have all the technology and capabilities to transform our world into a healthy global family. For each of us the work begins now, in our own home, by acting on our own personal truths and by educating ourselves to co-operate in the necessary planetary transformation.